ADHD to Clarity: The Chemical-Free Solution

Copyright © 2014 by Esmeralda Fox

Editors: Kimberly Rooks, April Miller, Christian Pacheco, Donna Melillo
Cover Design: 3-Sixty Design
Interior Design: 3-Sixty Design

Indigo River Publishing
3 West Garden Street Ste. 352
Pensacola, FL 32502
www.indigoriverpublishing.com

Ordering Information:
Quantity sales: Special discounts are available on quantity purchases by corporations, associations, and others. For details, contact the publisher at the address above.

Orders by U.S. trade bookstores and wholesalers: Please contact the publisher at the address above.

Printed in the United States of America

Publisher's Cataloging-in-Publication Data is available upon request.

Library of Congress Control Number: 2017948068
ISBN 978-0-9990210-2-6

First Edition

With Indigo River Publishing, you can always expect great books, strong voices, and meaningful messages.
Most importantly, you'll always ind...words worth reading.

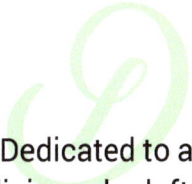

Dedicated to all who finally listen to Hippocrates, long considered the father of modern medicine, who left us sage advice: *"Let food be thy medicine and medicine be thy food."*

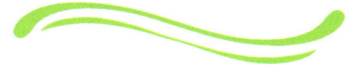

CONTENTS

ACKNOWLEDGEMENTS

This book has come about as a result of my healing. My hope is that others looking for a chemical-free approach of healing find encouragement and direction from my experience and guidance. I want to begin by thanking God.

This book and these recipes came so easily after learning to pray at Oneness University. Thank you Amma, Bhagavan, and all the staff at Oneness University for helping tens of thousands every year connect with the divine. This book could not have come about without you.

Special thanks to Dan Vega, Adam Tillinghast, and to all the staff at Indigo River Publishing for all your help and encouragement in the creation of this book. Your input has been invaluable.

Thank you Maritza, Eleonora, Jules, Yvonne, Svetlana, Magdalena, Michelle, Dena, and Liliana. Your friendship has enriched my life tremendously.

Love and thanks to my mother, Consuelo, for your help with the photography, for embracing my dietary and spiritual ways, and for incorporating them into your life. I loved watching you go from a size 12 to a 6 in a healthy way.

In loving memory of my father, Alvaro Quintero, whose numerous health concerns first caused me to question the standard American diet. Thank you for teaching me to love myself above all.

To my little sister and her spouse, Maritza and Matt, you both are my personal cheer corner. I take health to extremes sometimes, and you both have only love and admiration for me.

Love and praise to my greatest teachers, my constant companions, and my true loves: my husband, Zachary, and daughters, Sydney and Morgan. Thank you for being my recipe taste testers over the years. Your role in my life has served to make me my best self, and for that, I am eternally grateful.

PREFACE

I am thrilled to have found healing for my ADHD. This is not a term I use lightly, but that is the most descriptive word. I suffered for decades from hyperactivity, racing thoughts, impulsivity, and forgetfulness. I had mood swings. I was oppositional, irritable, and defiant. Getting along with anyone or getting anything done was routinely a stressful chore. New, healthy recipes coupled with a spiritual program that I learned at Oneness University healed me. I wrote this book at great expense to myself in hopes of sharing this message with those who find, as I did, that medication is not their answer.

If you have learning challenges or are interested in improving your emotional wellness, this book can help you tremendously. If you are looking to help another, such as your child, the book can also be useful. If you have another ailment, I recommend this book and the recipes within it as well. Nutritional deficiencies can manifest as illnesses. The reason they manifest as different illnesses is because each of us has a different set of genetic weaknesses, diets, and lifestyles. The information contained in this book helped me overcome ADHD symptoms. I know it can help others who experience a wide range of issues and ailments such as food cravings, anorexia/bulimia, diabetes, hypoglycemia, high blood pressure, arthritis, dementia, heart disease, fibromyalgia, demyelization issues, obesity, and more. How can that be possible? In general, our bodies require a diet that is low glycemic; high in protein, fiber, and minerals; and rich in enzymes (prebiotics), probiotics, chlorophyll, and oxygen. If you are looking to gain improvements in the areas of learning, beauty, physical health or mood, then please read carefully.

I have spent a decade reading about the nutritional value of food and the benefits of each nutrient. This book contains a compilation of recipes that deliver the highest nutritional value to your cells. In an effort to have these nutrients be well received, topics such as sleep, exercise, spirituality, and health in relationships are addressed, all of which comprise our LIFESTYLE. It is imperative to remove toxins from our environment. Environmental toxins are prevalent in the form of fluoride and chloride in our water, additives and preservatives in our food, antibiotics in our animal products, and chemicals in our toiletries, household cleaning products, and lawn care products. All of these create imbalances in our bodies and tax our liver and lymphatic systems, whose primary function is to remove toxins from our cells.

When I first began my journey, I was fortunate to be in a position where I could give my issues my attention full time. Otherwise, I might not have had the strength to endure. I have been relentless in my pursuit of results. In fact, you could call it an obsession. I know not everyone will share the same level of obsession as I did on my journey or invest the same time as I did. I realize change is very difficult. It requires time and effort you aren't sure you have. Life can get in the way. You have work, kids, studies, and other responsibilities that demand your time. In order to make it easier for you, I researched and learned everything I could so that I could then share it with you.

Remember, everyone is given the same twenty-four hours. Even if you start small, you will see your life change. Get up fifteen minutes earlier in the morning to convene with God or to meditate. Meditation allows me to connect with my own pain, the pain that comes as a result of everyday experiences as well as the deep rooted pain from my childhood. Every conversation with God brings me to new levels of self-realization, which translates into enormous benefits in my mood and behavior. Also, try a new, healthier recipe twice a week. You will start to feel better and be inspired to do more to change your overall lifestyle, physically and spiritually.

My experience of life improves with every emotional block that is removed via meditation. Thanks to God, I can be here for you. Feel free to contact me for a consultation. You can reach me at **EsmeraldaBFox@gmail.com**, or can visit my website at **ADHDHolisticSolution. com**. Alternatively, you can friend me on Facebook.

MY STORY

Our minds and bodies are machines that either function optimally or poorly depending upon what thoughts we keep and the diet and lifestyle we have. In my journey, I've found that learning what to eat and how to curb cravings for food allergens such as sweets, dairy, aspartame, nicotine, caffeine, molds, and alcohol needs to come first. A bizarre incident that makes this point is Dr. Alexander Schauss' investigation into a crime in which a man who had no history of criminal or violent behavior, committed an atrocious crime after being exposed to synthetic natural gas for six years. Dr. Schauss later wrote *Diet, Crime and Delinquency* in which he contends that in his ten years of working within America's penal system, "as many as 90% of all criminals show abnormal and altered body chemistry brought on by impaired nutrition and environmental assault." Information such as the data presented in Dr. Schauss' book has prompted numerous food experiments in juvenile delinquency institutions and jails. They all document dramatic drops in inappropriate behavior when common food allergens are removed. Dr. Julia Ross, author of *The Diet Cure*, echoes Dr. Schauss' findings by contending that a diet of junk foods or food allergens contributes to drug addiction by creating low levels in essential neurotransmitters, which regulate mood and affect behavior. I see this in my older self.

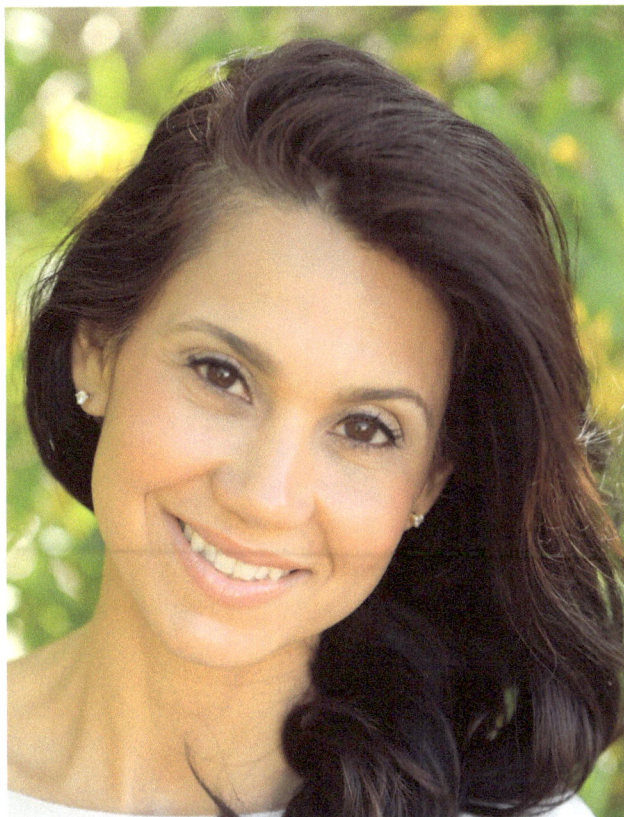

Growing up, my family and I ate the standard American diet full of plenty of cooked red meat, bread, milk, and desserts. Today, I see my old self as the know-it-all, loud, irritable individual with an interest in mischief that I was. I would get excited about new experiences and then grow bored and quit. In high school, I was on the forensics team and yearbook committee; worked at an ice cream shop, pizza parlor, and collegiate bookstore; volunteered as a candy striper at my local hospital; and was a lifeguard, all in my last three years of high school. I was never consistent with anything probably because obedience never gave me a rush. The only thing I didn't have in common with delinquents was that I never found myself in trouble, hard as I sought it.

*I resolved to be well naturally and
be an example to others.*

There came a point in my life when I no longer wanted to suffer from my aliments. I was serious enough to turn to medication. My illness was standing in the way of living a long, happy, and productive life. I went to the doctor and got a diagnosis of ADHD, followed quickly by a prescription. As I took the prescription, I found that I had more problems than I started with. I felt completely estranged from my children and had no chemistry with my husband. I prayed to a higher power. I resolved to be well naturally and be an example to others. I began to find information that helped me in that journey. The medication prescribed to me was part of a class of drugs called serotonin reuptake inhibitors, designed to increase the amount of serotonin circulating through my system at any given time. I then learned that foods like turkey, chicken, walnuts, and tart cherry concentrate contain tryptophan and melatonin, which also become serotonin in our bodies. Dr. Julia Ross's book *The Diet Cure*, which outlines how eight foods—sugar, gluten, dairy, corn, soy, caffeine, yeast and mold—create neurotransmitter imbalances, also seemed to fall into my lap at my local library.

I found that serotonin is a neurotransmitter that is produced and spread by neurons in the brain. It is formed by the amino acid tryptophan, a part of protein from our daily diet. Higher levels of tryptophan in the blood tell the brain to synthesize tryptophan into serotonin. Serotonin then helps to determine an individual's overall mood and to overcome mood changes, anxiety, depression, etc. Serotonin in the body helps to make one feel relaxed, happy, and confident. It also has many other uses, such as appetite control, mood and behavior regulation, cardiovascular function, sleep, muscle contraction, regulation of endocrinal secretions, memory, learning, and temperature regulation.

I was in so much pain because of my mood swings and racing thoughts, so I DECIDED TO DO SOMETHING RADICAL. I stopped all medications and adhered to a whole foods diet in hopes of finding true healing. I continued studying nutrients and the mind and put all my findings into practice. This has been no easy task, as I love dessert and processed foods.

My personal journey for healing inspired me to study nutrition, food allergens, supplements, neurotransmitters, right and left brain synchronization techniques, the power of meditation, positive affirmations, and personal development. Keeping my body well-nourished brought me to a new level of consciousness and eased my anxiety. I cannot emphasize enough the difference it made in my life. I did, however, still suffer from a racing mind and experienced a tremendous amount of tension in my body. I exercised aggressively but could not escape my hyperactivity. I thought these peaks and valleys were due to blood fluctuations, stones in my liver, sand in my kidneys, poor nutrition, distress in my visual system, and/or thyroid issues, but after addressing all these issues, I found some symptoms were still present.

Keeping my body well-nourished brought me to a new level of consciousness.

I've been Rolfed and hypnotized. I've done visual therapy, personal development, positive affirmations, right and left brain synchronization exercises, yoga, reflexology, acupuncture, and emotional freedom technique. I have recalibrated my nervous system using Feldenkrais movement. I have cleansed and nourished for nine long years and ate duck embryo for the stem cells. Through this, I improved. Certainly, I went in fewer circles than before in order to accomplish everything, but experiences in my world could still send my heart racing on average of about once a week. That was a huge improvement. But once a week or so, something silly like someone disagreeing with me, for example, triggered my fight/flight response, crippling me for about an hour. In that time, I was no longer capable of high-level thought and responses. I experienced tunnel vision, my hearing became muffled, my heart raced, and my mind screamed. It was awful. Inevitably, I would have to bring myself down, using deep duodenum breathing and meditation.

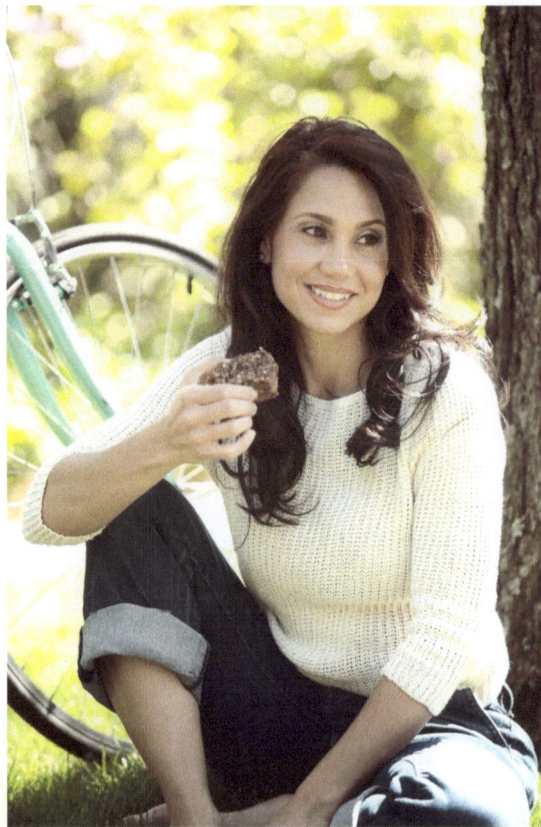

My ADHD was manageable because I could handle a panic attack. That said, I was present to the fact that ADHD was not completely absent from my life. I still missed some social cues that I would notice I had missed but only in hindsight. Listening intently to others was also taxing. I could only manage it for a short time before I became exhausted and irritable. Other times, my mind would fixate on a part of the conversation, and I couldn't let it go. I had to be vigilant, which still kept me from fully enjoying and relaxing into my life.

At this point in my recovery, I realized that I had recovered significantly but not completely. Years of research and sacrifice for this? So I prayed, and a couple named Bhagavan and Amma from Oneness University came into my life.

Oneness University is a school dedicated to teaching humanity how to ascend to a higher level of consciousness. I had tried everything else, and I wasn't willing to go back on medication, so I turned to God. I am very thankful to Amma and Bhagavan, the founders of Oneness University, for teaching me how to stay connected to God throughout my day to raise my overall level of consciousness. Today, I can honestly say that I no longer have ADHD, and I am so thankful. I spent ten years of going in a hundred different directions, only to learn what so many have said before: ALL ROADS LEAD TO GOD.

In that process, I became a certified wellness coach. I have 120 hours of training as a raw vegan chef, know and use Healing Touch and Reiki, am a Oneness Blessing Giver/ Trainer, and found God. Today, I both look and feel my best. I get to bed early and rise early, fully rested and ready to be productively engaged in my life, family, and community. My relationships and the quality of my life have improved immensely. My passion is sharing what I know and helping others bring their mind, body, and relationships to their peak state. I recommend that you get clear—CRYSTAL clear—about how things are going to turn out for you. Make your choice, and the path will be shown to you.

The good news is there is a solution to your issues, and eating naturally tastes good. The bad news is we are all addicted to processed food, and there is a certain amount of pain associated with this acceptance and recovery.

*Today, I can honestly say that
I no longer have ADHD.*

FOOD INTRODUCTION

Chinese medicine—5,000 years of wisdom—divides everything into a system of opposites known as yin/yang. Foods categorized as either extremely yin or yang are not conducive to meditation and emotional stability. The most yang emotion is anger and the most yin emotion is fear; they believe the two coexist. Extremely yang foods include red meat, hard cheese, and salt. Extremely yin substances include sugar, white bread, pasta, alcohol, and drugs. Diets high in these extreme foods bring on extreme emotions, and one creates cravings for the other. Eating too much meat brings on cravings for alcohol and sugar.

In the West, yin and yang food combinations are common. It's funny how they are often found together. Some common examples include spaghetti and meatballs, ribs and cobbler, burgers and beer or soda, chicken and linguine, steak and cheesecake, pizza and soda, eggs and pasteurized juice, and salted nuts and liquor. These foods have no fiber, rob our bodies of oxygen, introduce low-grade fats into our bodies, require large amounts of insulin to digest, send us on an emotional roller coaster, are congestive to the liver, and create large amounts of uric acid in the body, which stresses the lymphatic system and causes toxins to circulate.

Beauty is the physical manifestation of good health.

These recipes represent easy patterns to fall into and are difficult ones to discontinue.

These recipes also contain the common food allergens gluten, refined sugar, caffeine, eggs, cow milk, soy, corn, yeast, and molds. This world is clearly a buyer's beware. How strange is it that the eight foods that consistently and adversely affect the health and well-being of a significant portion of the population are on every television commercial, on every street corner, in mass quantities at every grocery store, and in vending machines everywhere? We are completely on our own in terms of health. This machine perpetuates itself via television, with its commercials about pharmaceutical drugs and processed addictive fast food. Healthy eating information is not part of the curriculum at school. There are no mainstream educational shows, commercials, or magazines that tell you how to be well naturally. For example, did you know that the processing of our sugar, salt, cooking oils, coffee, vinegar, juice, dairy, water, baby food and bread causes these foods to damage, not nourish, our bodies?

Healthy eating information is not part of the curriculum at school.

No one tells us that mayonnaise is rancid, table salt is bleached, white sugar is chemically processed, bread contains potassium bromate (banned in 100 other countries around the world), baby food contains low-grade sugar, spices are irradiated, shrimp is washed in chlorine, coffee is heavily sprayed with pesticides, gum contains an excito neurotoxin, cold cuts contain additives, cow's milk contains proteins that cause allergies, and in general all our food contains chemicals, sweeteners, food dyes, additives, preservatives, and fragrance. If you aren't feeling well, that's probably why. Instead, the message the machine perpetuates is that if you want to be well, you need to take a pill because your illness is genetic or can be managed through medicine. Often, there is not a single word regarding the role diet and lifestyle plays in our health. Anyone who says differently is deemed a health nut that has no credentials because he or she is not a doctor. It's very dismissive.

The truth is that regular consumption of these foods has a capacity to intoxicate us just as alcohol and any drug does. Today, so many of us are taking either a legal or illegal drug to get by. On every corner and even in schools, junk food beckons, and there is no education around this. We begin our days on the insulin roller coaster because eggs, pasteurized juice, and toast require a lot of insulin to digest. Even baby food contains sugar. These meals are full of common food allergens. Adults often add the stimulant coffee to this toxic mixture.

*We are slaves
to junk food.*

There are bake sales and candy vending machines for children and adults alike on every corner, and it is cheap and easy. The government uses our tax dollars to subsidize raw materials to produce processed foods, keeping processed foods cheap. This insulin coaster leads to violence (fear and anger) and drug and alcohol abuse.

We are slaves to junk food. Junk food creates sick people, delinquents, and addicts. Junk food also creates jobs within the fast food industry, the pharmaceutical industry, and in factory farms and a ton of trash. The delinquents employ the cops, judges, and lawyers and keep jails in business. The sick, which incidentally also include the addicts, employ the pharmaceutical industry, nurses, home aids, doctors, hospital staff, and health insurance companies. The plastic surgery industry also benefits, as does the vision and dental correction industries. This is the machine. Dr. Westin Price, a dentist who travelled the world studying indigenous tribes, was astonished to find people living in health and peace when processed foods were absent. In his book, *Nourishing Traditions*, he lists recipes for enduring health as well as his findings regarding the physical, dental, visual, and emotional health of these people. The machine we have in America isn't going to help us because it benefits from our lack of health, spiritually and mentally.

We must consider the world we create when we choose to live on this insulin roller coaster. We are never there for one another and are never sober enough to heal ourselves spiritually. If we all ate a whole foods diet, we would live in a very different place. Eating low glycemic is a step towards getting off the grid. Imagine that. How else can we participate in the world and within one another's lives? We must escape this slavery that keeps us all at constant odds.

Dear God,

I have become lost. I don't know how to engage my brothers and sisters, who I share this planet with, in a way that fills us all with your love and peace. Show me how to participate in the world in a way that lifts others and me to a higher level. Free me from my emotional roller coaster and fill my consciousness with the joy of the present moment. Give me eyes to see your ways so that I, too, may live in harmony with the Earth and all living things. Open my heart to the opportunity and prosperity in being in contribution to the highest self of others. I believe in my Father almighty, creator of Heaven and Earth, bring me close, rid me of the noise created by my sins, heal my broken heart and connect me fully with your magnificence. Strengthen me so that in difficult moments I might not despair nor become despondent, but with great confidence submit myself to your will, which is love and mercy itself. **Amen.**

EAT WELL, BE WELL

We generally want the highest quality in every area of our lives. We'll spend more on designer jeans, glasses, and handbags. Our automobile represents us, and our zip code defines us. These are the areas of our lives that we measure ourselves and that we work to improve. This is an invitation to bring that mentality to your diet and your spirituality. The thoughts we keep create our world. The foods we eat become the raw materials that create our brain, organs, and pleasure

Beauty is the physical manifestation of good health.

our everyday foods through healthy recipes, and a whole are not vine-ripened and many food miles on from other countries. and at the grocery in the loss of essential

The recipes in this that nourish without and lows that come because those highs are in beauty, physical health, Our bodies are machines. Just proper care and maintenance. Eat rich foods as you can, and watch the disappear.

hormones. Let us raise the quality of quality ingredients, new and foods diet. Today's foods freshly picked. They have them and often come Food ages during travel store shelves, resulting nutrients.

book contain foods giving us the highs with processed foods not free. We pay a price mood, and mental clarity. like any machine, they require as many nutrient-dense, mineral cravings, mood swings, and excess weight

So what types of foods and nutrients should you eat? Avoid foods that require large amounts of insulin to digest since insulin doubles as a stress hormone in the body, causes inflammation, and disturbs thoughts and emotions. The less insulin required to digest your meal, the better. Raw foods, incidentally, require less insulin to digest than do cooked foods because raw food contains enzymes necessary for digestion. High-grade sugars also require less insulin. High-grade sugars can also be referred to as oligosaccharides. Many do not require large amounts of insulin to digest and still nourish completely. Foods that are naturally high in oligosaccharides as well as protein include dark leafy greens, soaked seeds, soaked nuts, sprouted grains, beans, chicken, raw meats, fish, and eggs. You should also eat dense starches such as yucca, wild yams, green plantains, parsnips, turnips, chayote, red potato, and other root vegetables. Foods that create balance necessary for meditation include seeds, nuts, beans, grains, green vegetables, herbs, fruit, sea and root vegetables, and fish.

You are also looking to replace as many food allergens as you can with vegetables and seeds. The recipes found in this book are meant to help you find the healthiest foods missing from our everyday diets.

Our bodies are machines.
Just like any machine, they require
proper care and maintenance.

RAISING YOUR NUTRITION LEVEL

Today, many of us fall short of attaining our optimal health, a birthright. Yet when we realize that nutrients make our bodies function optimally and that the standard American diet falls short of supplying all essential nutrients our bodies require, our knee jerk reaction is to take supplements or self-medicate. That is thanks to the vitamin industry that has been diligently telling us the benefits of all their products. Today, the nutrition industry is a multi-million-dollar industry. We need to remind ourselves that our tongues long to taste, our teeth need to chew, and our system is set up to produce a bowel movement. The vitamins don't satisfy our rumbling bellies. We need to get full on the nutrients we require. What sense does it make to take a capsule of a healthy unrefined oil, such as flax seed, primrose, or cod liver and then fill up on low grade fats found in commercial salad dressings, ice cream, rich desserts, and mayonnaise? One vitamin capsule cannot give you what you need. It is not a magical cure. Instead, use superfoods. Superfoods are Mother Nature's multivitamin and provide far more benefits than vitamin pills, which are just synthetic chemicals. In the past, my reaction was, "I do have a good diet, but I'm not ever satisfied. I'm left with cravings." That's because I didn't use superfoods as ingredients, which offer a diverse and concentrated set of nutrients. Eat these foods until you are FULL on the nutrients your body needs for optimal health. Superfoods are foods with a high

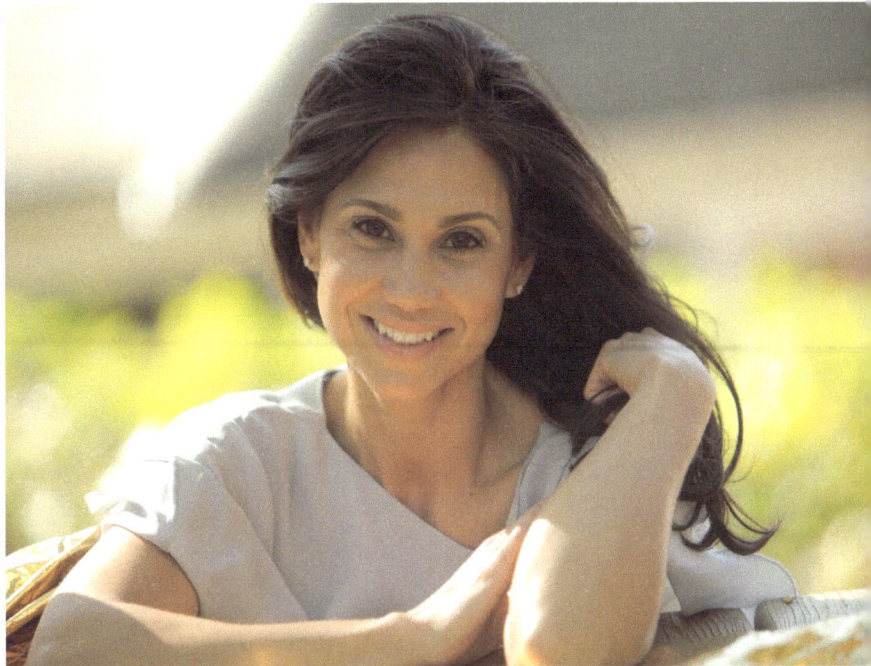

nutritional value within a small helping. Adding superfoods to our recipes is essential to healing our bodies and getting rid of cravings for processed foods. It ensures that we get the nutrients we require while adding flavor, fiber, enzymes, and texture to recipes that incorporate them.

Below you will find some superfoods found in my recipes. All of these ingredients can be purchased online. So many ask me why my diet is so complicated. They are curious about Shan Zhu Yu and what the seeds floating around in my breakfast cereal do. To that, I say that we all have weird things in our diet. Those ingredients in processed food are just as strange—stranger even. Please do your own research on the nutrients below. Add them to your diet. The superfoods below keep me balanced and away from processed foods that we all seem to accept and crave with addiction.

Nutrient	What is it?	Used In
Shan Yao, Shan Zhu Yu, Ling Zhi and He Shou Wu, Maca, Mesquite	Herbs famous for helping us to make a powerful antioxidant superoxide dismutase, a class of enzymes that repair cells and thus help with aging. Naturally high in iron, zinc, and alkaloids, they are known to nourish the endocrine system, increase energy, and enhance health.	Brownie, smoothie and coffea recipes
Lugol's Solution	Iodine, found in shellfish, is essential for thyroid function and digestive health. I encourage you to consume shellfish on a weekly basis. If you do not, then consider using Lugol's Solution. FYI, too much iodine is as dangerous as too little iodine, just a drop will do.	Mylk and smoothie recipes
Chlorella	Dense green nutrient helpful in evacuating heavy metal and other toxins from the body.	Brownie and coffea recipes
Bee pollen/royal jelly	Substance that contains amino acids, carotenoids, phytosterols, fatty acids, and enzymes for improvements in overall health.	Cereal recipe and nut mylk recipes

Continued

Nutrient	What is it?	Used In
Chia, sunflower seeds and other seeds	Food high in essential fatty acids, antioxidants, vitamin E, and protein, making it capable of nourishing the brain and nervous system.	Cereal recipe
Camu camu and amla	High concentration of naturally occurring vitamin C and more bioavailable than synthetic versions. Vitamin C protects the body against oxidative stress.	Brownie and nut mylk recipes
Spirulina/any bluegreen algae/chlorella	High in protein, calcium, vitamins A, C, and D, and essential amino acids.	Brownie recipe and basmati rice
Raw cacao powder/nibs	Natural source of antioxidants and magnesium.	Cereal and brownie recipes
Raw agave/raw coconut nectar/yacon syrup/fresh pressed sugar cane/raw local honey/black strap molasses/mesquite & lucuma powders/dark stevia	Whole food sweeteners that nourish the body and contain high concentrations of vitamins, minerals, enzymes, chlorophyll, soluble fiber, antioxidants, proteins, and other health supportive compounds that are known to stabilize blood/sugar levels.	Low glycemic desserts and breakfast recipes
Spices/herbs	Ingredients that improve the digestibility of most foods and add another dimension to our foods in terms of nutrition and flavor.	Meats and vegetables recipes, as an alternative to seasoning packages.

Continued

Nutrient	What is it?	Used In
Fruit pulp/concentrate	Frozen fruit pulps can sometimes be found without preservatives. Making your own juice allows you to avoid the chloride and fluoride and allows you to cut back on sugar, raise the quality of your sugar, and raise the quality of your salt.	Juices
Aloe vera	Plant that contains over 200 active components, including vitamins, minerals, amino acids, enzymes, polysaccharide, and fatty acids.	Smoothies and nut mylks
Butter oil/cod liver, coconut, walnut, almond, olive & other unrefined oils	Unrefined oils are fats and are essential to the proper functioning of our nervous system, brain, and hormones. Oils have a freshness date and become rancid 6 months after opening.	Dessert, raw green sides, and cereal recipes.
Colostrum	Colostrum contains an abundance of nutrients, including growth factors, lipidic and glucidic factors, oligosaccharides, antimicrobials, cytokines and nucleoside. It is rich in immunoglobulins which are certain types of protein involved in promoting the immune system and fighting germs.*	Substitute for commercial cow's milk in our everyday diet
Eggshell/pearl	Highly bioavailable source of calcium. Commercial edible pearl comes ready to use perlcuim.com.	Boil organic eggshells 30 seconds and add to nut mylk recipe
Sea minerals/fulvic acid/shilajit/food grade diatomaceous earth/bentonite clay	Minerals that are essential nutrients in the body that catalyze many functions in the body such as the manufacture of insulin. Minerals have become deficient in our soil and diet. Mineral concentrates attempt to increase the number of minerals in our diet for improvements in overall health.	Great addition to smoothie or vegan mylk recipe
Berries: goji, mulberry, blueberry, cranberry, etc.	Food naturally low in sugar but high in vitamin C and other antioxidants and cleans and nourishes our bodies.	Great addition to any cereal or dessert

Continued

Nutrient	What is it?	Used In
Ashwanandha, Bacopa, Mucuna, Maca, Gotu Kola, Lucuma, Reishi, Moringa, He Shou Wu	These herbs nourish/support the body at a cellular level	Good way to consume is as a morning coffea

* Robert K. York, M.D. author of *Colostrum, A Journey Toward Better Health and Brighter Tomorrows*, describes how fibromyalgia rendered him incapable of continuing his medical practice, how he found no help in traditional medical treatments for the disease, did research on his own, discovered colostrum, and through it got his life back.

Your recipes, as the recipes in this book do, should contain the nutrients needed, in quantities required to satiate your appetite. A diet that is high in superfoods such as foods containing sulfur like apples, eggs, bok choy, Brussels sprouts, broccoli, and cauliflower deposit the raw materials we require to make insulin and muscle as well as deposit necessary fiber into our diet. My bok choy salad recipe adds this essential food into our diet in a way that is delicious. The lasagna contains cauliflower in a way that you'll love. Adding superfoods specifically is an amazing diet tool, so please see chart above. Super oods such as but not limited to food-grade diatomaceous earth (the exoskeleton of insects, a pure form of silica) keeps food cravings away, evacuate toxins, strengthen our bones and teeth, and in general keeps our organs and glands fully functional. Consuming an ⅛ tsp of diatomaceous earth is sufficient to curb our appetite and give energy. Please consume with a full glass of filtered water, as its tendency is to slightly dehydrate. Raw foods have a different role in the body. Raw foods such as raw fish, eggs, and red meat add l-tyrosine into our bodies and well as essential enzymes. Tyrosine is a neurotransmitter that acts as energy. Raw animal product is another way to increase the amount of nutrients present in dinner and to curb cravings. Those who find themselves unable to control their appetite might find that consuming only raw foods for a period of time to be very healing. Please see my meat tartare and other raw recipes. Dessert syrups from berry concentrates instead of sugar and vinegar give us large amounts of antioxidants that heal our nervous system and keep our brain functioning optimally. Finally, the coffea recipe introduces herbs that are full of essential minerals and antioxidants often missing from our everyday diet. Even the brownie recipe, made from whole foods, seeks to nourish. These are the healing recipes Americans need.

Superfoods are
Mother Nature's multivitamin.

SPIRITUAL AND MENTAL HEALING

Stuck negative emotions and fears can be just as toxic as chemicals to our psyche because they keep us aligned to our lowest consciousness and are often responsible for internal disturbances and self-destructive behaviors. For this reason, my program includes the Oneness Awakening Class as a means of addressing and discovering our inner world. The Oneness Awakening Class is a non-denominational class that helps to release embedded emotions by using the help of the divine for improvements in all relationships, especially the relationship with oneself. As per the teachings of Amma and Bhagavan, noise within our minds is a symptom of fears and pain trapped in our body and unconscious mind. Gaining freedom from your pain and anger—which is no one's fault but simply the state of man—is a gift from the divine, and it is available to every living being who asks to be liberated. Whenever you experience a negative emotion, call to God and ask to be liberated.

A large part of my program includes prayer because, invariably, there are moments when you find yourself stuck and need to overcome your pain. Prayer is simply a conversation between you and your divine power. You can do it anytime and anywhere. It can set you free from the pain and suffering that comes from everyday interactions that adversely affect your health.

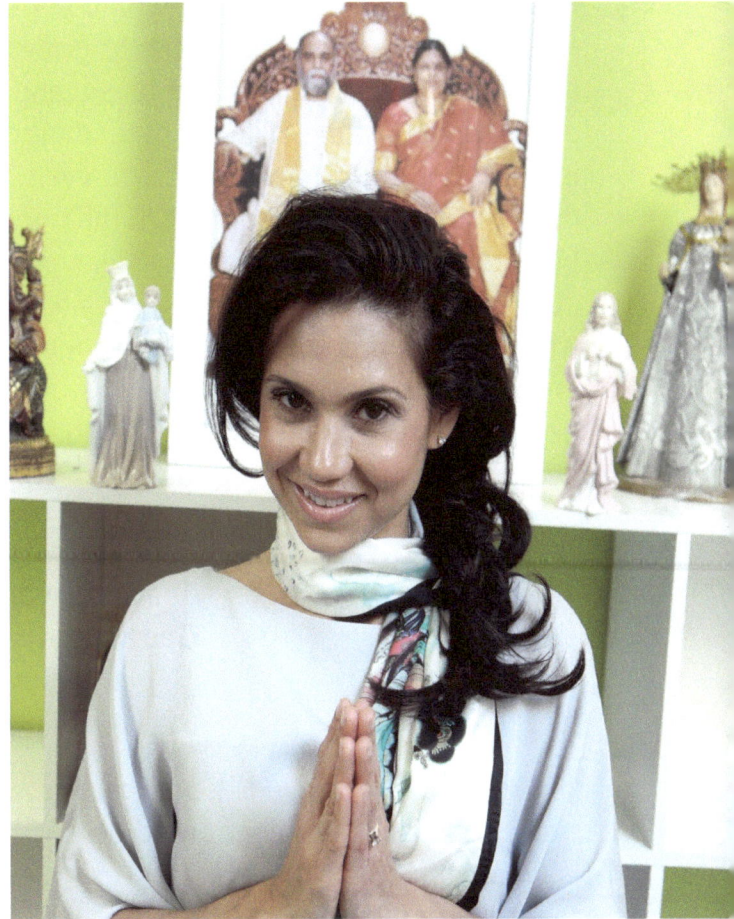

The simple act of convening with God can dramatically change the experience of your life. After each shift in my consciousness, I will watch in awe as my experience of a situation changes. For example, I noticed I'm less bothered by taunting. The person who taunts has not changed, but my experience of being taunted has. Once my new, more pleasant reality becomes old, I am ready to grow again. My mind races less and less every time I do this. My restlessness is reduced, and peace, joy, and harmony come into view. These shifts happen in the stillness of meditation. I sit quietly and share an experience with God in which I confront my issues. We even laugh at my pain together. I fully experience any dysfunction without judgment. In that moment, I understand my level of personal evolution. I am not as advanced as I would like to be, but I realize that where I am is beautiful. In the stillness, I can hate and like my pain. I experience a full range of emotions associated with my dysfunction: frustration, anger, numbness, and then acceptance. Once I accept my situation and take responsibility for it, I can make a new choice regarding what kind of experience I would prefer. I say (to God or to my highest self), "Let's have the experience of being in the moment as opposed to being in a rush."

The simple act of convening with God can dramatically change the experience of your life.

I recommend you sit and meditate. It's called evolving the self, and it pays off tremendously. When confronted by my illness, I convened with God and meditated. This is what worked for me. To discover your inner world, ask yourself questions like, "What is the most confronting experience in my day? What prospect made my heart race today?" Making quiet time daily can reduce the amount of emotional baggage you carry and thus keep you from using food in an unhealthy way. The teachings at Oneness taught me not to blame, only to experience every relationship fully and to become aware of how I am feeling when I think of loved ones. If discomfort is there, I have learned to look closely. A heart to heart with God brings healing.

Right now, I'm working with God on control issues. I say to God, "Please help me to allow as opposed to control." I've begun to see how I don't like surprises. I thought it must be something deeply hidden from my view. As I convene with God, I see how fearful I am of the unknown. I control out of fear, and it affects every area of my life. I have purposefully made my world small to avoid surprises. I keep others at a distance because they are unpredictable. My body is very tight and inflexible, and my blood pressure is so low it scares my doctor.

The opposite side of my control issue is my impulsivity, which catches others off guard, is unpredictable itself, and surprises both others and me. It is the opposite side of the same coin. My issues with impulsivity created awe-filled situations for me. To overcome an unpleasant personal characteristic, I generally try a million things in the area of behavior modification and nutrients for mental clarity. Eventually, I come back to the discipline taught to me at Oneness wherein I accept that I cannot help myself and that I need help from the divine. Then, I sit down. I breathe. I address my divine and say. "Look at this. I constantly do this, and I don't like the results. I promise myself not to do it again, but then I do. I disappoint myself. I annoy others, and it creates adverse situations. Please, God, help me." Afterwards, I just wait and notice how many more times impulsivity rears its ugly head in my life. Each time I see it, I just notice.

Each new experience of my impulsivity teaches me something about myself. For example, my impulsivity impairs my ability to work with others in a way that is pleasurable and beneficial for all. It has been so difficult to ask for help because I am also very arrogant. I believe I can do it myself, I don't trust, and I am controlling. How can I receive from the Lord? It's been difficult to be open to help from the divine, but the world has seen to it that I find myself in situations where I have no choice but to surrender. Personally, this experience has been painful. The benefits, however, have been extraordinary.

Prayer brings about healing, and healing relationships with our parents, spouses, and children have a powerful effect on our physical and emotional health. We are all connected and can, therefore, help one another. I regularly notice behavioral changes in the members of my family when I bring God into a stressful exchange. Other times, I sit quietly in front of my photo of the Lord and look back on an unpleasant exchange with my spouse, child, or family member. Each conversation with God shows me how my behavior and/or personality traits create situations for me. I am at times the perpetrator of the very behavior I am complaining about. My prayer is to be set free of such exchanges.

I recommend you sit and meditate. It's called evolving the self, and it pays off tremendously.

Call God to your aid whenever you experience any negative emotion. I wasn't getting on well at home, but I had a great desire to keep my family together. I reflected, I prayed, and help came. So find a character flaw or negative recurring experience that is present in you. Notice how it lowers your quality of life. Then, you can focus on it in prayer. Don't give time and other resources to negative emotions. If you do, you will find yourself doing things out of hurt. The passing of time will bring you bitterness as opposed to joy. Instead, take time to fully experience whatever stresses you and makes you scream and want to fight during prayer. That's when I let my emotions run high. I feel and experience issues quietly with God. Then, I pray for freedom to the Lord with passion. My prayer might sound something like this: "I just cannot go on this way. Teach me a new way. Do not leave me like this." This prayer can be three-minutes or three-hours long depending on what feels right at the moment. When the student is ready, the teacher will appear. In the end, I thank God. I get excited about the new level of harmony that has entered my life.

Optimal wellness is when we reach a point so peaceful that we seek adventure by going after a dream rather than being busy with drama or seeking the highs found in a fight or thrill-seeking behaviors. When we can be truly present for others, especially our family who require our unconditional love, we are well in every sense of the word.

We cannot find the joy in life when we are distracted by the roller coaster created by cravings, arguments and illness.

You cannot be free until you see that, so ask for a guiding light around your issue. Remember to stay present. Wait to see what part you play in the drama that affects you. It will come. This is what I learned at Oneness University. Keep an eye out for new levels of harmony so that you thank God when you see it. I stay vigilant. I look to see changes in my own behavior around the issue I prayed about. Is it gone? Is it still there? Just notice. Don't judge or stress. Just watch. One by one, my negative emotions have been lifted, and I know prayer and the help I received during the Oneness Awakening Class is the reason.

Many people have shared stories of recovery just like mine. Our stories all seem to have one thing in common. We acted with faith and enthusiasm. I was convinced that there was an answer and that I had found it. At one point, I declared I was healed and began teaching and writing for magazines. Without realizing it, I made use of a law in the universe: "ACT AS IF AND YOU WILL BECOME AS IF."

There are so many studies regarding the power of the mind. I have now fully recovered from adult ADHD, a rarity. Yet if you research recovery, you consistently find that it's the mind (or God) that does it. Somewhere in the mind lies the most powerful force known to man. I was so happy every time I learned of a nutrient that would bring me to the next level of health. I kept measuring and celebrating every time I noticed any improvement in my ability to concentrate, participate in a long conversation with another, stay calm, and experience joy. I think it was all this celebrating, gratitude, and deep belief that kept healing each ailment I wanted liberation from. Keep your eye on the prize, and you too will reach your goals. Healing takes place when you choose to recover today as opposed to a distant point in the future. Equally important is the consumption of nutrient- and mineral-rich foods, avoiding common food allergens, drinking plenty of water, exercising, and sleep.

Join me in being present to the level of joy you are capable of. For me, it's been relatively low for much of my life. Focusing my attention there has created a shift in the relationship I have with others and the one I have with myself. Putting your attention on your inner world can create shifts in your relationships and improve the quality of your life.

WHAT YOU SHOULD KNOW

At one point in my life, I was eating lean chicken breast and brown rice, switched to egg white omelets, used skim milk in my boxed cereal, and cut my desserts by a third. I couldn't figure out why I still was not getting any better. Evidently, I was eating the wrong foods. As previously mentioned, we need nutrient-dense, mineral-rich foods free of common food allergens. What do I mean by nutrient-dense and mineral-rich? It means adding foods like sprouts, soaked seeds, sustainably raised/grown vegetables, herbs, unrefined oils, and superfoods loaded with antioxidants.

Beauty is the physical manifestation of good health.

There is a silver lining in all this news. Our bodies are not difficult to understand. Our bodies essentially require fats, sugars, antioxidants, and mineral salts to thrive. Our bodies are hardwired to look for and love these life-sustaining substances. Any danger that arises out of that hunt comes when our food moves away from its natural form.

Let us look at what these life-sustaining substances do in our bodies:

✦ Oligosaccharides or sugars in the body are most like the language of the body. Each cell is bathed in an oligosaccharide structure across which all cellular communication takes place.

✦ The fats we consume build our brain, nervous system, skin, cell walls, and hormones. Those are the bricks and mortar that build the structures where our memories and thoughts are housed.

- Salt contains minerals that act as the ground for all the messages in our bodies since our bodies' cells communicate via a system of electrical impulses.
- Finally, there is water, the medium that our bodies need to exist. Every cell requires a certain amount of water in order to carry out regular cellular activity. Without water, cells could not maintain their integrity (shape) nor could they transport nutrients and toxins. Water is life.

Let us now look at what is available in terms of nutrition from the standard American diet and what we ought to be eating instead:

Oligosaccharides: Low-grade sugars such as refined sugars and carbohydrates oxidize the collagen on our faces, causing premature wrinkles. They deplete us of mood stabilizing nutrients, melt muscle off our bodies, and leach calcium from our bones. Refined sugar and artificial sugars become the oligosaccharides that our bodies use to create cell structures, across which cellular communication takes place. The ability of cells to communicate properly then begins to decline. That usually spells disaster. We have so many names for these disasters as each disease has a different name.

Our bodies are not difficult to understand.

Our tongues long for a satisfying sweet taste. That's when cravings begin. We eat brownies and cookies full of those low-grade sugars such as aspartame, chemical and alcohol sweeteners, and white sugar to satisfy our tongue. These sugars spike our insulin levels and do not nourish. Aspartame can be found in soda, gum, breath mints, and more and is considered an excito neurotoxin because it seeks out brain cells and kills them on contact. The reason our tongues love the taste of sweetness is that sweetness tells us our food is ripe and ready to eat. Farm-fresh produce that is sweet means that the food has nutrients that are bioavailable to us. As we move away from gardening and toward grocery stores, our vegetables are picked before they are ripe. They are instead flash ripened in a synthetic fashion, and our tongues know the difference. The same sweetness is not present. It is no wonder we wince and crinkle our noses at the thought of eating our vegetables and crave low-grade sugars instead. What can we do— become gardeners? That is so labor-intensive. How could we find time to do anything else if we garden? The general consensus here is we simply can't. So we think we have no choice but to leave gardening to the professionals.

The truth is there is a way. I love the movie *Back to Eden*. I started my first ever garden after watching that film because it made gardening seem possible for me. In this educational film, Paul Gautschi urges us to cover our garden with wood chips. Wood chips absorb and release rainwater in massive quantities, keeping the soil moist so that people don't need to water and can instead rely completely on rain water. In addition, wood chips create a healthy medium for the plants to grow in, deleting the need for fertilizers or pesticides. Your earthworms will thrive. It keeps soil soft by releasing gases so that you don't have to till, and the covering keeps weeds at bay, all of which cut back on the labor associated with gardening. If you fear getting termites from the wood chips, consider using food-grade diatomaceous earth. I implore you to watch and start your own garden. If mosquitoes and other insects are an issue, plant marigolds or lavender or look into the benefits of using diatomaceous earth.

*"There is nothing more powerful
than an idea whose time has come."*
–Victor Hugo

27

It is time we change our minds about having a garden. We plant and water decorative bushes, shrubs, and trees at great expense. Consider an edible garden instead. The city plants trees and shrubs with taxpayer dollars. Why can't they be fruit-bearing? How much fun would it be to decorate our homes with a garden that is edible as well as ornamental? Processed foods can never compete with wholesome food. Our kids would prefer an apple to a sugary snack if the apple were fragrant, hydrating, sweet, accessible, and full of the nutrients their bodies require. Plant a fruit-bearing tree today and take wellness into your own hands. The alternative is to continue depending heavily on grocery store produce.

Fats: You must put in an effort to find good and life-sustaining fats because the fats currently in our refrigerators and restaurants—salad dressing, mayonnaise, ice cream, cookies and other sweets—are rancid. A significant percentage of our bodies are made from fat, so any balanced meal must contain fatty acids. Fats are vital to our survival, and the longing in our bodies for fats is actually a survival mechanism. Healthy fats that clean our arteries and livers can be found in soaked nuts and seeds, avocados, coconuts, fatty fish, sheep and goat dairy, and unrefined oils. Part of any satisfying meal has to consist of fats in order to satisfy our bodies' requirements. The recipes in this book show you how to incorporate healthy fats into your diet. The more healthy fats you add to your diet, the fewer cravings you will have.

If you travel regularly and are forced to depend on restaurant food, making your own salad dressing and dessert is one of the easiest ways to increase the quality of your meal because remember that the fats currently in our refrigerators and restaurants —salad dressing, mayonnaise, ice cream, and other sweets—are rancid. I carry a small bag in my purse when I travel. I carry three dates, a few carob chips and/or raw cacao nibs, a small shaker of sea salt, and two types of unrefined oils in a small capers jar. The oils are olive oil and a sweeter oil like pecan, almond, walnut, or sesame oil. In warm climates, coconut oil is an acceptable choice. The olive oil is primarily for salads and dinner while the sweeter oil is great for converting any fruit salad into a satisfying dessert. When others order dessert, I order fruit and then add salt, sweet oil, my carob chips/ cacao nibs, and dates in order to create a healthy and satisfying dessert.

Salts/Minerals: Today, many of us have mineral deficiencies that adversely affect our health. We often do not realize how fragile our bodies are. Our thyroid gland is particularly vulnerable to mineral deficiencies. When our thyroid functions optimally, we have energy, our skin glows, our hair looks full, our cholesterol is balanced, and our sleep patterns are healthy. We can regulate our body temperature and have a healthy weight.

Minerals like iodine, which is found abundantly in shellfish, keep our thyroids functioning optimally while synthetic minerals, such as chloride and fluoride, compete with calcium, another mineral, for absorption into our bones. Not only do they lower our calcium absorption, but chloride and fluoride also yellow our teeth and cause health concerns, according to Dr. Joseph Mercola, a New York Times best-selling author, osteopathic physician, and proponent of natural solutions for better health. Fluoride damages your sleep/wake cycle by calcifying our pineal gland.

For good health, drink plenty of filtered water.

Our planet used to naturally filter all our water.

These toxins can enter our bloodstream through our skin when they are used in our swimming pools and in our drinking water. The regular use of chloride bleach in laundry and cleaning is adversely affecting our bodies. To prevent those toxins from being adsorbed through our skin, we should use food-grade hydrogen peroxide in our laundry and pools, and unless you have well water, you need a whole-house water filter. Install a point-of-entry water filtration system so that your bath and drinking water are free from chloride and fluoride. If you are having sleep issues, especially if you are using sleeping pills to compensate for your damaged sleep/wake cycle, then drink an ounce of tart cherry concentrate two hours before bedtime. Tart cherry concentrate is high in melatonin, which will help you to sleep. Furthermore, melatonin can be manipulated by the body to make serotonin, which has been shown to improve our sleep cycle. A proper diet provides the serotonin you need without having to add supplements.

For good health, drink plenty of filtered water. Our water is different today, affecting our overall health and well-being. Our planet used to naturally filter all our water. Our water had minerals from being pressed with force through rock, had ozone from being hit by lightning, and was oxygenated by the crashing waves. Now those substances are not present. Know that these changes, even drinking filtered water, already stress our bodies. We don't need to take the extra step of consuming carbonated drinks, which deposit large amounts of sugar and carbon dioxide into our systems, depleting us of oxygen. We are low on oxygen as it is.

Chasing Ice is a documentary released in 2012. James Balog uses time-lapse photography to tell the story of global warming. Research conducted on the ice glaciers tells the story that over the past 800,000 years, the amount of carbon dioxide in the air has been between 180,000 and 280,000 parts per million. The present is the first time in history where the levels of CO2 have reached 400,000 parts per million, and it is rising fast. Carbon dioxide is the waste product the animals and we put off, and I don't need to tell you that we all need oxygen to breath. Otherwise, our brain cells begin to die within one minute. It's safe to say that anything that depletes our bodies of oxygen further and deposits carbon dioxide into our bodies is dangerous.

In order to put back some of the minerals missing from our water, add fulvic acid/ trace mineral concentrate to smoothies and nut mylk recipes. Natural supplements like fulvic acid, sea vegetables, and trace mineral concentrates help us to re-mineralize our bodies to improve our dental health, bone health, and mental clarity. Consume high-quality sea salt, really only Remond's salt or Hawaiian black salt, which is local to the U.S. We don't need to import our salt. Raw salts, as a mineral, add minerals back into our everyday diet.

Salt contains approximately 92 minerals in quantities so tiny they can barely be measured. These minerals are essential to the functioning of our cells, and these minerals need to stay in balance with one another in order to catalyze processes within our bodies. Iodized table salt is the most processed salt on the market, and you'd be surprised how much table salt is found in processed foods. The more processing salt undergoes the fewer nutrients it contains and the more addictive it can be to consume.

Like Himalayan and Celtic salt, sea salt is not processed and is considered a whole and raw food. Our bodies have a natural intelligence that becomes disturbed and enters into an addictive, dissatisfying relationship with a substance when the nutrients our bodies expect are not there. How else can we explain how we can eat an entire bag of salted potato chips or popcorn at the movies and not be satisfied while a mouthful of salt water at the beach, without realizing it, satisfies completely our salt desires? It's because table salt is very processed while ocean salt contains every last mineral, leaving us completely satisfied before we have had too much. I recommend Redmond's Real Salt because it is a high-quality domestic sea salt.

Salt contains approximately 92 minerals in quantities so tiny they can barely be measured.

Salt is also very important for the body because it is the ground for messages in our bodies. When we sweat excessively or exercise, we lose salt. Pay attention to your body's cravings for salt, especially after heavy exercise, so that you do not find yourself craving processed foods.

As I went on my journey to mental, physical, and spiritual health, I began to see why so many of us are sick. I saw why the foods we eat play an enormous role in our longevity. Studies from countless universities and independent researchers have well established that as fact. Below is information that can put you on the optimal nutrition path to experiencing a sense of well-being you never thought possible. The following information is bulleted so that it can be more easily referenced. If you are struggling in the area of physical health, mental health, emotional health or experiencing premature aging, you will likely find solutions if you act on the following information.

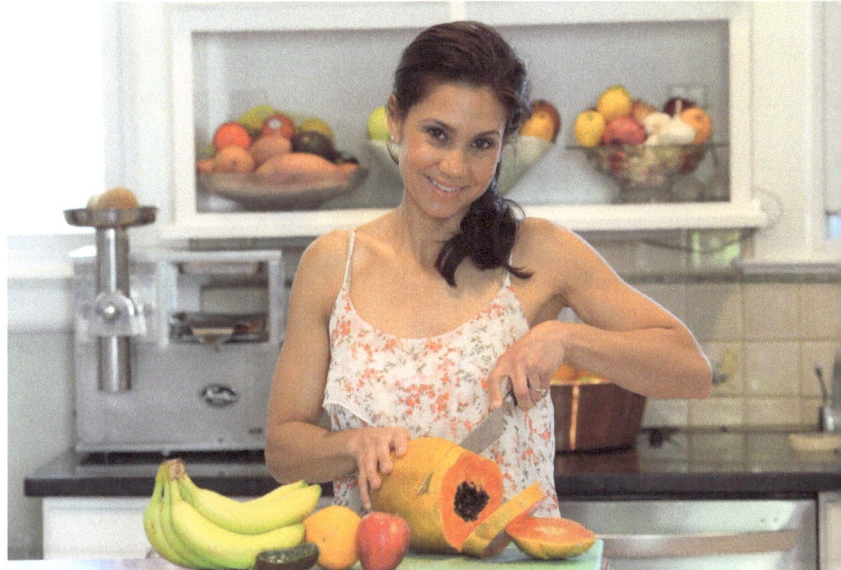

+ ADHD, depression, and mood swings can be helped significantly when we add mood stabilizing niacin (vitamin B3) and essential energy enzyme CoQ10 to our diet. These nutrients are needed in abundance by many but are deficient in our everyday diet. Tobacco plant leaves are very high in both and very helpful for balancing our moods and cholesterol, which improves mental recall capacities and cardiac function.

I recommend you grow a small tobacco plant indoors. Seeds cost $.99. Plant seeds inside a seed starter tray that comes with growing pellets. Seed starter trays come in 50 or 72 pellet trays and can be purchased any time of year at your local hardware store. Water with warm water, and keep them near a sunny window. Once you have a tiny plant, about an inch tall, eat it in your salad twice a week. This should give you a huge boost. In the winter, you might need a grow light. I plant a few seeds in a pellet on a weekly basis so that I always have new sprouts growing. You can do this and avoid buying synthetic forms of the nutrients you require.

- ✦ Blood sugar stability equals emotional stability, which is a topic you can find more of in Criminologist Dr. Alexander Schauss' book *Diet, Crime and Delinquency*. Consuming a completely satisfying and nourishing meal that requires little insulin to digest is the name of the game. Filling up on fish, sprouted non-glutinous grains, raw greens, beans, fruits, salad sprouts, and vegetables as much as possible is the best way to keep our bodies strong and minds clear. Some people choose to eat raw meat, fish, and eggs while others prefer beans and grains. Either is fine as long as you avoid processed foods. Gymnema Sylvestre and green stevia (not the white stuff that is bleached) are the herbs that also healed my body of low blood sugar.

- ✦ The eight allergens I have mentioned before—gluten, refined sugar, caffeine (including chocolate), soy, dairy, eggs, molds and yeasts (leavening, peanuts, vinegar) and corn—adversely affect the body. . If you are not the picture of health, delete these for a year and see what happens. Allergens are also brought on by additives, preservatives, artificial sugars, food dyes, fillers, bleaching agents, and anti-caking agents common in processed foods. Chemicals in our laundry detergents, lawn care, toiletries, perfumes, pet care products, hair care products, and make-up and nail supplies can also adversely affect health with allergens. Both Dr. Feingold and Dr. Rapp found that such foods and chemicals could cause not only a physical symptom such as a rash but could also affect emotional wellness and/or mental clarity. As such, an allergic reaction to a food or chemical could manifest as moodiness, sleepiness, or brain fog and often causes us to hold on to five to ten pounds of excess weight.

- ✦ Each fruit, vegetable, green leaf, and grain of salt—in a word, all whole foods—contain all the nutrients our bodies require to digest it. When foods are fried, milled, preserved, pasteurized, homogenized, frozen, canned, dried, or colored, they lose nutrients. Make time to prepare food as opposed to opting for something out of a package.

✦ Redundant protein, usually from eating too much red meat, causes vitamin B deficiency. Too much cooked red meat can tax and deplete our bodies' vitamin B reserves. Vegetables, sea vegetables, fruits, beans, greens, chicken, fish, and sprouted non-glutinous grains are high in B vitamins that are essential for a stable nervous system. There is much research that shows that B vitamins can be a natural treatment for mood and learning challenges. Make an effort to delete bread and fill up on other foods. You can also eat meat raw so that you can get what you came for in as few ounces as possible. I'll elaborate on that more.

✦ Not eating enough fish can be harmful. Omega 3s are vital for healthy brain function, and having too much red meat adversely affects the proportion of omega 3, 6, and 9 that should be present in our bodies. Omega 3 nourishes the brain and helps with learning and vision. It has been shown to have a positive effect on dyslexia. Consuming fish and shellfish on a weekly basis not only adds iodine, zinc, and omega 3s to your diet, but it also fills you up. With at least two meals a week of fish, you can avoid red meat and the omega 6 and 9 that is contains.

Consuming a teaspoon of fish oil every other day is also recommended. Cod liver oil is high in omega 3 fatty acids, vitamin A, vitamin D, and CoQ10, which is an essential energy enzyme for proper functioning of our heart and liver. To counterbalance the increase in mercury that invariably comes with more fish in your diet, be sure to have chlorella as food staple. It is easily found at any health food store. You can add a ground tablet or teaspoon to any smoothie you have during the week, to nut mylk, or to your hot chocolate or coffee.

✦ Grains containing gluten can damage your digestive system, and can weaken your immune system. Consider deleting grains from your diet. How about using plantain flour for all your baking needs? For a significant percentage of the population, weight gained from grains appears as flab or rolls that give a dough-like appearance, meaning there is no muscle in that fat.

- Cow's dairy has been linked to anemia, high cholesterol, asthma, and mental imbalances. If you constantly crave pizza, macaroni and cheese, sundaes and you notice dairy is in everything you eat, consider the possibility that you have become allergy addicted. Do yourself a favor and read *Milk: The Deadly Poison* by Robert Cohen. *Don't Drink Your Milk* by Doctor Osaki and articles by Dr. Mercola further point to why dairy from cows is not the perfect food. Thousands of children get tubes in their ears because of tremendous mucus build-up caused by the casein found in cow's milk. Replace cow with sheep and goat dairy before considering surgery.

- Caffeine causes a spike in our blood sugar levels, giving us false energy. Instead, you could consume raw fish and raw organic beef, which are high in l-tyrosine. L-tyrosine is the neurotransmitter our brain naturally makes to feed our adrenal and thyroid glands and to give us energy. This route is much better than consuming the caffeine that beckons on every corner.

- Issues with high cholesterol, heart problems, and high blood pressure abound in this country. Myriam Ehrlich Williamson warns of the dangers of fluctuations in blood sugar levels in her book *Hidden Dangers of Insulin Resistance*. Dr. Richard and Karilee Shames, authors of *Thyroid Power*, explain that high cholesterol despite a good diet is symptom of low thyroid. Low thyroid often goes undiagnosed and is the culprit behind a myriad of health issues. Keeping your thyroid healthy begins with keeping blood sugar fluctuations at bay. *Escape Fire*, a documentary that exposes the perverse nature of healthcare, informs us that the leading cause of death among those with blood sugar fluctuations is heart failure.

If you crave sugar, then eat the real thing. Press your own sugar cane. Sugar cane is a seasonal food, but a conversation with the gentleman who stocks the vegetables at a local Latin/ethnic grocery revealed that sugar cane be ordered upon request all year around. I press sugar cane by peeling the outer peel and then use my Norwalk juicer to press the juice. You can look on YouTube for videos before buying any machine to see how that machine works. You need to use the most powerful machine you can afford to get the best results. One glass of fresh, pressed sugar cane blended with an ice-cube-sized piece of peeled aloe vera creates an extremely nutritious food combination.

+ Did you know that refined sugar depletes you of the brain chemicals that give you a strong sense of well-being and stabilize your appetite? If you have issues with food cravings, anorexia, bulimia, mood swings, OCD, hypoglycemia, diabetes, anxiety, or obesity, then listen closely. Heavy amounts of sugar are the first mind altering substance we consume and is considered to be a gateway drug. If your cravings for sugar are completely out of control, you could benefit from drinking fresh, pressed sugar cane juice or learn about free-form amino acid therapy in Dr. Julia Ross's book *The Diet Cure*. You can also make desserts another way. See my recipes or purchase a book on raw desserts. For a subtle change in cooking habits, sweeten your homemade cakes by grinding pitted dates in a coffee grinder with the flour. That sweetens the flour and helps you to avoid white sugar.

+ PMS is generally considered progesterone deficiency. Premenstrual appearance of migraine headaches, anxiety and states of confusion, dizziness, clumsiness, and even suicidal tendencies are part of this syndrome. The Creighton Model brings this information to us. This model is NaProEducation technology, a form of natural family planning approved by Christian churches that is found to be 99% effective. Family planning without the hormones sold by the pharmaceutical industry is real. Strange how the industry fails to inform us about natural solutions. Of course, the answer is obvious. They wouldn't make any money selling natural cures. Progesterone builds bones and repairs brain cells. If you have PMS, your body is trying to tell you something. Balancing your hormones begins with a lifestyle that is low stress, low glycemic and has abundant sources of fatty acids.

+ Did you know that cavities are an infection near your brain? They are very dangerous. Tartar quickly accumulating on your teeth is indicative of a poor state of physical health. Modify your eating habits. Look into oil pulling and avoid fluoride. It's easy enough to keep unrefined sesame oil in your shower. Swish a tablespoon full around in your mouth for ten minutes while you wash and dry. This oil will attract bacteria that you can then spit out. Fluoride we get at the dentist, in our water supply and pools, on all non-organic vegetables, and in beverages such as coffee, beer, juice is a chemical as opposed to a fluoride that is naturally present in sardines and vegetables. Dr. Mercola speaks out against the heavy use of the chemical fluoride in this country. Search to learn more.

+ Foods such as dairy, sugar, molds, yeasts, carbonated drinks, pasteurized juices, and dried, salted, or high-glycemic foods and animal product cause congestion and deplete oxygen in our bodies, causing an imbalance that manifests differently for each of us. A diet and lifestyle high in chlorophyll, unrefined oils, clean water, aerobic exercise, antioxidants, and sprouted seeds nourish and oxygenate our bodies. Oxygen in our bodies supports the proliferation of good bacteria, supports our immune system, and keeps infection and illness away. If you have acne, brain fog, anemia, cancer, or autoimmune issues, this diet can increase the quality of your life. Information about baking soda, ozonized water, and chlorophyll for cancer helped me to realize the importance of oxygen in the body. To keep up your oxygen levels, drink seed mylk, use goat and sheep dairy products, and make water your favorite drink.

+ Eating fresh foods as opposed to frozen, canned, fried, and pulverized foods like bread and pasta gives us a range of nutrients, such as chlorophyll, probiotics, enzymes, water, fiber, and minerals that feed us on different levels and awaken our naturally joyful, creative state. CoQ10, for example, is found on the outer shell of grains, which is lost in the milling process. Choline in eggs is lost during cooking—a great reason to make your own mayo. In *The Diet Cure*, Dr. Julia Ross reminds us that hundreds of studies confirm the rancidity of commercial mayonnaise and salad dressings. She goes on to explain that soybean, safflower, canola, and corn oil are very fragile oils that become rancid before they are even bottled and are dangerous to our health. Please read labels to see what your favorite products contain.

HEALING OUR BODIES ONE AILMENT AT A TIME

Food: Superfoods and Raw Food

For me, mood swings and brain fog were my biggest complaints. Criminologist Dr. Alexander Schauss and Dr. Julia Ross, a pioneer in the field of mood and behavior and a specialist in the treatment of eating disorders and addiction, found that a diet of refined foods causes changes in mood and behavior. My research has revealed that the liver and pancreas work together to keep our blood sugar levels balanced. Regular consumption of high-insulin meals weakens this mechanism, causing blood sugar levels to fluctuate. Fluctuations create eating disorders, cholesterol issues, other health concerns, and mood swings. The mood swings can be severe, bringing on violent or suicidal tendencies, but it can just as well be subtle, creating irritability so that we are unable to be kind towards those around us. The cure for this is something I've already explained: consuming a diet that requires little insulin to digest.

Superfoods such as Gymnema Sylvestre, green stevia and He Shou Wu have powerful capacities for regulating blood sugar levels. The first time I took them, it was 6 a.m. and right before my commute and class. Lunch was at noon. At around 11 a.m., I felt a

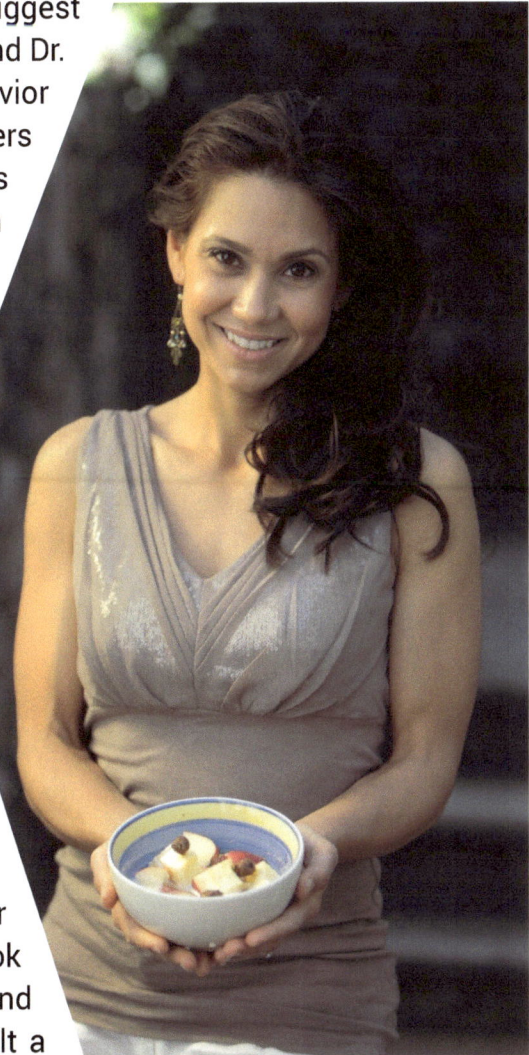

coldness coming into my body like I had felt many times before, drawing my attention away from the lesson. Then, almost immediately, I felt a warmth travel through my veins, and I was able to concentrate again. I used these intelligent nutrients for over a month, all the while I felt they kept the floor from dropping out from under me. The He Shou Wu (fo-ti), a substitute for coffee, remains in my diet because it keeps neurotransmitters alive. To learn more about fo-ti, you can go to http://hyperionherbs.com/shop/he-shou-wu-extract-16-oz/ on the web.

A diet that is at least half raw keeps many ailments away.

A diet that is at least half raw keeps many ailments away, not just fluctuations in blood sugar levels. That information is what motivated me to make arrangements so that I could attend an intensive one-month raw food preparation program at 105 Degrees Culinary Academy, located in Oklahoma City, Oklahoma. We barely had any raw foods in our diet previously, and I knew that information would take my family and me to a higher level of wellness. Raw food classes taught us to sprout seeds, nuts, beans, grains, greens, and herbs and prepare fruit, sea vegetables, and green vegetables in a way that awakens their enzymatic value, giving us a whole range of nutrients missing from our everyday diet. Raw foods are naturally nutrient-dense and mineral-rich because they contain live enzymes that contribute to the assimilation of nutrients as well as deposit healthy bacteria into our bodies. Consuming enough enzymes and natural probiotics is possible when we incorporate raw foods into our diet and cut back on cooked foods that can leave our bodies without the enzymes necessary for that optimal assimilation of nutrients.

Some raw foods also contain more nutrients than their cooked counterparts, as is the case with green vegetables, herbs, oils, sugar, salt, fish, red meat, eggs, animal dairy, fruit juice, vinegar, sprouted seeds, and nuts. Having a diet that is half raw and half cooked increases your level of wellness by facilitating absorption of nutrients. People who have weakness in their pancreas find support in a diet that is at least half raw. Please remember that raw fruit is not the answer because of the amount of natural sugars they contain. Sprouted foods and thinly sliced vegetables are a solution. My raw fat burn salad, raw coleslaw, raw greens, spiralized zucchini, cereal, smoothies, salad dressings, brownie, and nut mylk recipes can add raw foods into your everyday diet in a way that is easy and delicious. I encourage you to try raw foods and make them part of your diet. Have a raw dish with every meal.

Some raw foods also contain more nutrients than their cooked counterparts.

Handling foods that are raw with care will ensure that you get the benefits while avoiding becoming sick. Please notice that when sprouting, I've asked you to place a few drops of food grade hydrogen peroxide into the water to kill mold. Please do not skip this step because a moldy sprout is poison. A half-gallon-sized mason jar is ideal for sprouting because it allows excellent ventilation of your sprout, thus minimizing mold. Raw fish and red meat should be fresh and organic and preferably free-range or wild. Use your sight, smell, and touch to verify it is fresh. Marinate your red meat or fish immediately, portion it into serving-sized pieces, and then freeze it. When you are ready to eat, thaw your portion in cold water and consume. This helps to reduce the amount of bacteria on your food prior to consuming.

Water

Water is also a great healing substance. Dr. Batmanglidj, author of *Your Body's Many Cries for Water,* recommends halving your body weight and consuming that number of ounces of water daily for optimal health. For example, someone who is 160 pounds

41

should drink 80 ounces of water daily. Batmanglidj's short paperback is packed with information regarding how consuming plenty of water helps the body to create energy. A fully-hydrated system creates plenty of digestive juices and helps the body to avoid digestive issues. Water in our joints acts as shock absorbers, keeping bones and cartilage protected—especially in our spinal column. The discipline of Yoga views spinal health as the fountain of youth. Dehydration also reduces the amount of blood in circulation, stressing our heart and so much more. I'm sure after you've read his book, you will find a tremendous amount of respect for water.

Urine

Now, the next healing substance can be such a controversial topic, but as a wellness coach, my job is to investigate everything. Urine is a miraculous healing substance that is free and available to everyone. I mean, who doesn't urinate? And given the saying that the best things in life are free, then maybe urine is the best? We are taught that urine is a waste product when, in reality, our bodies create 28 liters of liquid nutrition daily that our cells can use, and it's sterile. One-and-a-half liters gets excreted as part of a safety mechanism daily, allowing us to over-consume sugar and salt and not die. The other 26.5 liters become our blood as well as the amniotic fluid we were all created in. Urine is filtered by the most intricate filtration system known to man: our own kidneys.

Keeping our livers healthy is another step in creating a healthy body.

Fresh urine can be used on our skin to clean an open wound. It won't burn. Urine is the only skin cleanser and moisturizer in the world that can penetrate the various layers of the skin, clean away dead skin cells, and fully-hydrate the skin. Urine contains nitric oxide in abundance. Nitric oxide was named Molecule of the Year in 1992, by both the journal *Science* and the American Association for the Advancement of Science. If ingested, the low-weight molecule nitric oxide in urine helps to evacuate toxins stuck in the cells, prevent thrombosis, lower blood pressure, increase powerful anti-blood-clotting properties, eliminate plaque stuck in the arteries, and optimize circulation, including penile flow contributing to erection. Fresh urine also contains nutrients in readily available form, kills parasites by boosting the immune system, and provides the body with antibodies for illnesses it has been exposed to, thus stimulating healing.

To learn more, read books on urine therapy. I encourage you to leave no stone unturned when searching for optimal health. The best way to use this life-giving substance is to keep your insides clean so that your urine does not repulse you. A couple of recommendations are staying fully hydrated or blending a piece of pineapple and a peeled lemon or lime (and as far as I'm concerned, if it's organic and you have a high-powered blender, keep the peel). Then, drink it. This makes your urine taste better. Recently, I'm in love with food-grade diatomaceous earth, which also keeps urine clean (as mentioned), curbs appetite, and makes skin glow. Diatomaceous earth is a natural form of silica that our bodies need. It is very inexpensive. I paid $25 for 10 pounds.

Nitric oxide and antibodies are concentrated in morning urine. Collect more than an ounce of urine from midstream and drink it within 10 minutes. This is considered fresh urine. If it stinks, consider what that is saying about the state of your body. None of us need a Ph.D. in medicine to know that the fouler the odor from our body or its fluids, the further we are from health.

Cleanse

Keeping our livers healthy is another step in creating a healthy body and curing our ailments. Cleansing the liver will help with a number of issues and ailments. The liver is the organ that processes fat in our bodies as well as creates hormones to regulate our endocrine system, digest our food, and regulate our blood sugar levels along with hundreds of other processes. Our livers can become overwhelmed with toxins, affecting our mental clarity as well as the liver's ability to function. Some of us do not process vaccinations very well, and residue from childhood vaccinations along with pharmaceuticals, additives, preservatives, food dyes, and other toxins remain trapped in the liver. Large amounts of cooked animal product, present in the standard American diet, have been known to create protein balls that clog our livers. Our livers are a system of ducts that, when congested, cannot properly secrete the enzymes the body requires.

Supporting the liver begins with consuming fresh as opposed to rancid, processed, preserved, and heated oils—essentially consuming a good type of fat. Consuming unrefined oils or oils with a freshness date—such as coconut, walnut, sesame seed, pecan, olive, hazelnut, hempseed, borage, evening primrose, flaxseed, red palm, fish, cod liver and butter oil—as well as fresh fats found it avocados, salmon, sardines, fresh soaked nuts, and seeds gives our bodies high-grade building blocks to create our brain, nervous system, and hormones, which are all made up of fat. Dr. Weston Price found that butter oil has tremendous nourishing properties, and when mixed with cod liver fish oil, its properties escalate to exhibit medicinal properties. These fats also help to cleanse the body of unhealthy fats and "bad" cholesterol and keep our liver and arteries clean.

A clean liver and body create a healthy heart, clear vision, and clear thought.

Regular care and maintenance of our liver as well as our intestines, kidneys, lymphatic system, and other organs require that we participate in regular cleansing. A clean liver and body create a healthy heart, clear vision, and clear thought. A liver flush recommended by Andreas Moritz in *The Liver Flush and Timeless Secrets of Health and Rejuvenation* is helpful in clearing stones. *Cleanse and Purify Thyself* by Richard Anderson is another good source for a liver flush recipe, and the benefits of cleansing are stated in the book.

Once a week, I recommend you begin your day with ¼ cup of unrefined olive oil and 2 tablespoons of fresh-squeezed lemon juice to cleanse your liver. Another favorite liver cleanse is pineapple and peeled lemon blended in ¼ cup of filtered water and consumed once or twice a week. For more information, read *Timeless Secrets of Health and Rejuvenation* by Andreas Moritz.

In an effort to ease the burden on your liver, read up on green cleaning or natural cleaning. Our liver has the task of removing all the chemicals from all our toiletries, laundry detergents, lawn care, household cleaning, nail care, car deodorizers, carpet chemicals, and more. All of these chemicals are toxic and need to be evacuated. In general, we could use baking soda and vinegar for cleaning all surfaces and castile soap for dishes, laundry, and our bodies.

Similarly, getting rid of heavy metals in your body is a way to increase your level of health. Heavy metals in the body adversely affect a host of physiological processes in our bodies. Heavy metals are found in bread, antiperspirant, lip balm, skin cream, make-up, baked goods, vaccinations, aluminum disposable cookware, vehicular emissions from leaded gasoline, fertilizers used in agriculture, and aluminum pots. In short, they are found everywhere. It is so easy to have too many heavy metals in our system. Anything that touches our skin ends up in our blood stream, and all of these toxins contribute to poor health. There are even diets that call for removal of chemical-laden toiletries for weight loss. Cook in stainless steel, cast iron, or other high strength metals, while avoiding Teflon and aluminum. Foods such as chlorella (an algae found in tablets or powdered form) and cilantro help evacuate metals. If you suspect you have a metal toxicity, you can also research home screening tests to see if one is appropriate for you.

CHANGES CAN BE CHALLENGING

The foods we eat become our brain, hormones, and organs. When we increase the quality of the raw materials our bodies use to create itself, we experience improvements in beauty, learning, mood, physical health—basically in every area of our lives. The problem is that junk food is addictive and found in abundance everywhere, especially if you live in the city or in a low-income area. Fast-food restaurants prey on the weak, and avoiding all this unhealthy food takes resolve, a commitment to be well, and practice.

This change is not easy for any of us for various reasons:

✦ Our favorite family memories are tied to our favorite dishes.

✦ We have sugar loving parasites, which crave sugar.

✦ Processed food is everywhere.

✦ Habits are hard to break.

✦ These foods give us pleasure.

✦ We do not know better.

✦ We like the flavor.

It is so much easier for us to do what we've always done, what we are familiar with, and changing for the sake of changing doesn't work. We need to have a reason to change. What are you after? Yes, a healthy diet can help you in every area of your life, but that's too vague. You need to make your reason personal so you have the strength to go on when complacency inevitably rears its ugly head. Creating a new habit requires an expenditure of energy and vigilance so that we don't fall into old habits that keep us stuck. We can't forget that sweets are easy to come by and that they are tasty. We need a reason that matters enough that we put those sweets back when temptation hits and you begin to wonder why you are avoiding sweets.

Finding relief from an ailment, for one, can be a powerful motivator. When I first began my research, I knew I was sick and tired of being sick and tired. I needed to find a cure for my ailments. I proceeded to make changes in my diet and lifestyle, while keeping my goal in mind and keeping my resolve. It is so important that you do that as well. Draw a connection from your diet and lifestyle to your physical and emotional health.

If your reason for change is to be beautiful, that's your body's way of wanting health. BEAUTY IS THE PHYSICAL MANIFESTATION OF GOOD HEALTH. Glowing skin is a manifestation of a clean liver, oxygenated blood, and healthy fats. All of your organs are working to keep your brain functioning at its highest potential. The state of your liver determines the amount and quality of blood your heart and brain get. Clean, oxygenated blood gives life and vitality to the brain and skin.

Finding relief from an ailment, for one, can be a powerful motivator.

How the fats we consume sit on our body are a manifestation of the quality of our brain, nervous system and hormones. A tight waistline is indicative of digestive and hormonal health, while thyroid dysfunction can manifest as a sagging throat, sagging skin, and grey undertone. In so many ways, beauty is the physical manifestation of good health. When you admire beauty, you are admiring health.

Getting clear on what your specific, personal reason is will give you the strength to change. Choose the one you feel strongest about and keep it ever present.

Here's what you should do:

- Create that connection in your mind between an unhealthy food and your most nagging ailment.

- Have an alternative food.

- Create a plan and work that plan. Write down your everyday food like bread, pasta, dessert, and cereal and create a food you will eat instead. Begin by substituting a food a week.

Here are some replacement foods/tips you can use to get more nutritional value out of a meal:

✦ Use seed and nut mylk with your favorite cereal.

✦ Use cacao nibs instead of chocolate.

✦ Enjoy steamed sweet potato with butter oil and sea salt to help curb sugar cravings.

✦ Keep warm soup in your home to snack on in the winter.

✦ Snack on low-sodium toasted pumpkin seeds.

✦ Snack on fat burn foods, such as radishes in water with dash of sea salt and twist of lemon/lime. For a full list, see my Fat Burn Salad recipe.

✦ Add black beans to your brownies or make my Raw Brownie recipe.

✦ Grind pitted dates with your flour in your coffee grinder to sweeten your baked goods.

✦ Make your own baked goods and use non-aluminum baking soda and powder.

✦ Make the Egg Punch recipe instead of scrambled eggs now and again.

✦ Experiment with free-form amino acids (see The Diet Cure).

✦ Make a raw apple or fruit pie at home.

✦ Prepare your fruit using my Spiced Seasonal Fruits recipe; it's a great quick dessert.

✦ Sprinkle soaked chia seeds into your cereal and water bottle.

✦ If you drink alcohol, add B-1 & non-flush vitamin B-3 to your diet.

✦ If you fry, upgrade your oil to red palm and olive oil. The ratio should be 1:5, respectively.

✦ Make yucca and plantain fries. Both are considered anti-inflammatory and cut down on grains and chips.

✦ Add fiber such as chayote, cauliflower, or yellow squash to your lasagna to cut back on cheese while adding fiber and nutrients.

✦ Replace spaghetti with spiralized zucchini in your spaghetti dinner dishes to add chlorophyll, fiber, and enzymes to your diet.

- Begin your day with three glasses of water.
- Substitute avocado for cheese and commercial mayo in your sandwich to cut back on rancid fats.
- Prefer whole foods to supplements. Use cod liver oil as opposed to vitamin A or D vitamins. Eat amla or camu camu rather than vitamin C made in a lab. Vitamin E supplements can be replaced by frying and sautéing food in that combination of red palm and olive oil mentioned above. Tart cherry concentrate can replace melatonin and sleep aids. Replace raw meat/fish for caffeine. They are naturally high in L-tyrosine, an energy neurotransmitter. Eggshells are a great source of calcium.
- Prepare your greens raw so as to avoid destroying the chlorophyll present in your precious food.
- Use butter oil on your toast, thus increasing the amount of vitamin K present in your diet.
- Vary your milks. Goat's milk is high in B-12, while seed mylk is rich in zinc.
- Put the contents of your sandwich on a salad, and cut back on bread.
- Make soups using a wakame broth on occasion to vary your soup bases.
- Sprout on a weekly basis. My favorite sproutable foods include buckwheat & whole oat groats and broccoli sprouts.
- Add pumpkin seeds (pepitas) that have been soaked for one hour to your guacamole.
- Add raw vegetables to soups and beans.
- Prefer my homemade cereal recipes and similar recipes to commercial cereal as often as you can.
- Add sprouts and/or sesame seeds to rice.
- Seed crust recipes can replace glutinous crust in all your dessert recipes.
- Substitute oxygen-rich water for carbonated drinks as often as you can.
- Press your own juice; delete pasteurized juice from your diet as much as you can.

- Cardamom seeds or cloves replace aspartame-laden breath mints.
- Those high-cholesterol sundaes are easily replaced by a sliced banana/plantain, walnut oil, dash of salt, cacao nibs, and berries.
- Vary your morning coffee by using my coffea recipe.

Sit down and figure out what food you want to replace and create a plan for what you will do instead. If you have an alternate food and create a plan, then you'll always have a replacement in mind and a game plan when that complacency is there. When you think of _____ (an unhealthy food, i.e. cookie, cake, ice cream), you will reach for _____ (your substitution). When you get home from _____ (work or school or somewhere else), you usually reach for _____ (an unhealthy food), and that food is being replaced by _____ (a healthy option). When you watch TV, you eat _____, and your new healthy option is _____. At night, I snack on _____, and your new option is _____. And so on.

You can also replace eating unhealthy foods, especially for comfort, with pampering yourself instead. When you get home from a long, hard day, you could take a warm bath, get a massage, read a chapter in your favorite book, get in a steam bath, go for a walk, call a friend, or whatever treat you can think of instead of going for that unhealthy food.

Also, make it a point to add new and healthy recipes one at a time into your repertoire of foods. It is okay if that takes a year. Many people eat the same dozen recipes over and over. Expanding these introduces new nutrients into your body and awakens new areas of your mind so that positive new thoughts that will serve you can emerge.

Make a commitment to have sprouted seeds or raw greens in your diet at least once a week, and then increase the commitment to twice a week. The junk will push itself out naturally. Go at your own pace, and be kind to yourself. Know that nothing is wrong in the world and that every moment is just right. Never judge yourself.

Also remember that sometimes it's what we don't eat that keeps us healthy. If you need to fill up on yesterday's leftovers, that is fine. too. There is a spark that is present in people who eat well. Along with a healthier diet, there are a couple of lifestyle changes that will make a difference.

Sleep

Sleep is another powerful way to keep our bodies balanced. I recommend getting to bed by ten o'clock at least three times a week for improvements in ADHD symptoms and health. Getting to sleep by ten o'clock keeps your body working optimally. As per Chinese medicine, the liver has a cleansing cycle that is skipped on evenings that we are not lying down with lights out and eyes closed by ten o'clock. Suzanne Somers, author of numerous health and wellness books, explains that our bodies regenerate hormonally only at night. T.S. Wiley in *Lights Out* explains that the brain interprets light at night as fear, which affects our nervous system adversely. Her research shows that the most restful sleep occurs in the dark of the night. Only in complete darkness can your body completely clear away stress. Getting to bed by ten o'clock allows you to sleep for seven hours prior to sunrise. Dawn diminishes the quality of your sleep. Her recommendation is to sleep in the darkest room possible by covering alarm clocks, night lights, alarm system lights, and anything that gives off light in an effort to sleep more fully.

Other points to consider are our bodies are more susceptible to electromagnetic fields while we sleep. Please put your phone on airplane mode, unplug large appliances near your bed, and keep a piece of orgonite near your bed. Orgonite is a combination of crystal and metal that is known to balance energy. Orgone energy was discovered by Dr. Wilhelm Reich in the 1930s.

The internet is a great resource for learning about orgonite and for purchasing it. Orgonite can be purchased for as little as $15, a very small price to pay for protection from harmful electromagnetic frequencies. I trust it, and I recommend it to you. Tart cherry concentrate is a natural source of melatonin, a sleep inducing hormone.

You can purchase 8-10 ounces by Dynamic Health online for $10. Magnesium can also help us relax more fully. Nuts are naturally high in this nutrient, so enjoy nut mylk. free-form amino acid 5-htp and vitamin B-6 is another great sleep aid combination that can be purchased at a vitamin store or online.

11-Minute Duodenum Breathing

ADHD is also an imbalance of the fight/flight response. High- level emotional intelligence can only take place when the nervous system is stable. Our nervous system is divided into the sympathetic and parasympathetic nervous systems. When our fight/flight parasympathetic nervous system is active, we are anxious and defensive, as opposed to being in listening, learning, and digesting mode. Being present and emotionally available occurs when our fight/flight system is off. Otherwise, we are jumpy, impatient, bored, or in need of action and adventure. Action and adventure are wonderful, but imagine trying to parent when all you want to do is go. Exercising from 5 a.m. to 6 a.m. helped me to be relaxed enough to help get my children ready for school in the morning, as did deep breathing when I needed to be calm.

To do duodenum breathing, inhale deep into your lower abdomen and allow it to inflate as you say "Sou" in your mind. Exhale by contracting your lower abdomen and forcing the air out while saying "Hum" in your mind. The inhale begins to happen automatically as you contract for the exhale. This eleven-minute exercise calms the mind and slows thoughts. I also do this while I drive, listen to another person, while worshipping and especially when I feel confronted because my mind constantly wanted to be running at a thousand miles an hour. This gave my mind something to do so that I could get a little peace.

Exercising

Exercising can be an example of deep duodenum breathing. This type of rhythmic breathing is exactly what you need to assimilate all the nutrients you take into your body, release toxins from every cell, oxygenate your brain, and use up your ATP at a cellular level, thus jump starting cellular activity as well as building muscle and bone. Basically, exercise is life. Exercise is healthy when done to the point your body can handle. Don't push yourself to exercise to the point of sleep deprivation or requiring stimulants, steroids, energy bars/goops as this is counterproductive.

Support Groups

Just because ADHD is your disease to manage doesn't mean you have to go on this journey alone. There are several outreach and support groups for those battling this illness. Band together, share your stories, and lift each other up!

GROCERY LIST

We have become accustomed to purchasing the same things over and over. When you go to make my recipes, you might find that you don't have what you need already, and that can be very frustrating. I don't want that to happen to you. You are going to need to make changes in what you purchase and keep in order to shift to this diet. When you look around in your fridge, you probably make sure you have bread, eggs, milk, yogurt, cheese, jelly, salad dressing, and cereal, you see? Then, when you go to prepare things, you have what you need.

Please keep the following around so that you can make these recipes:

✦ Keep natural supplements such as spirulina, bee pollen, cacao nibs, mesquite, fo-ti, berry concentrates (pomegranate, blueberry, cherry concentrates), walnut oil (or other sweet unrefined oil), unrefined olive oil, and fish oil around. Changing your diet needs to begin with addressing your cravings for tobacco, caffeine, aspartame, and stronger substances like drugs and alcohol. The reason you take these unhealthy substances is because your body chemistry is out of balance. free-form amino acids also exist in nature and can be found in those natural supplements. Getting them into your diet immediately will help you transition to a healthy diet with ease.

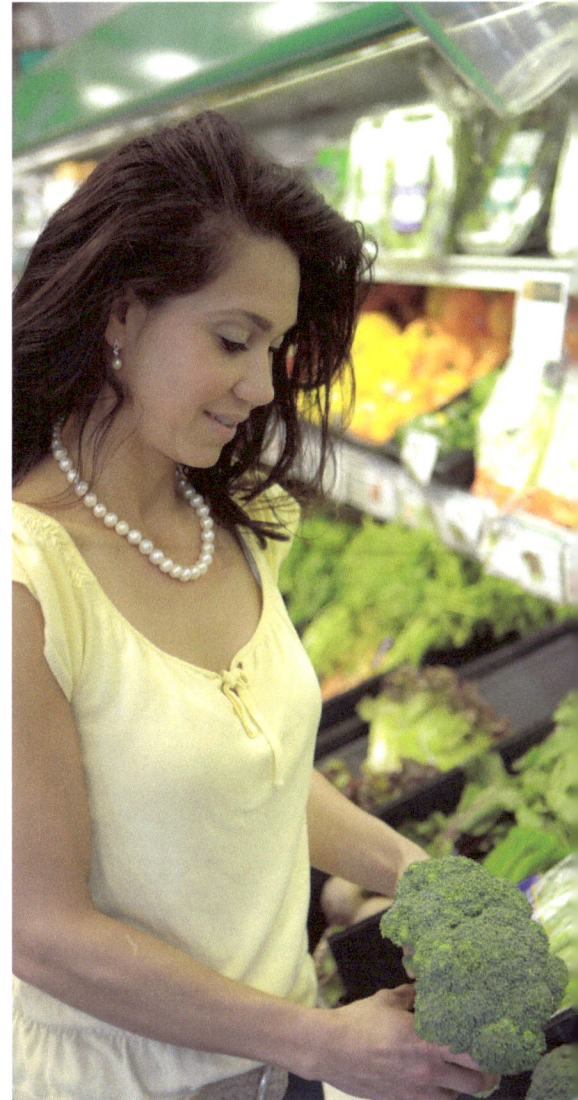

✦ Keep nuts around to soak. You are going to need soaked nuts as a source of fat because you are cutting back on eggs, salad dressing, and dairy. Since nuts take an entire day to sprout, it's best to keep soaked nuts in your fridge at all times. Doing so will make any recipe in this book easy to make. Recommended nuts include walnuts, almonds, pecans, hazelnuts, and macadamia nuts. Please do not use peanuts or cashews. In a pinch you can use seeds, as they only require one hour of soaking and still contain the fat, enzymes, fiber, and nutrients like zinc that nuts bring to our diet.

Nut preparation

✦ Soak for eight to ten hours at least, preferably all day.

✦ Allow your nuts to drip dry in a colander for an hour.

✦ Place nuts in an open plate to dry for 8-10 hours or overnight. Cover with a colander/sieve to keep safe from pests.

✦ Place nuts in a container in fridge.

✦ To avoid work, you can purchase sprouted, raw, unpasteurized nuts online.

Please note that the shelf life is one week.

When soaking almonds, discard any almond that floats as these are rancid and could be harmful to your health. Keep your raw nuts in the fridge at all times, and look for a freshness date when purchasing them because nuts are only good for one year from the date they are picked.

Keep prepared nut mylk or some goat milk around. Being able to reach for milk anytime is a convenience we have all become accustomed to. Always having nut mylk or goat milk in your fridge will ensure a similar convenience. This book contains excellent nut mylk recipes you can use.

Keep raw, shelled sunflower and pepitas (pumpkin) seeds in your freezer. Since their soak time is one hour, these can be ready to go anytime. Soaked sunflower seeds, chopped apple, amla and berries makes a wonderful cereal. This is my cereal of choice. It is really satisfying.

Keep dates, powdered amla (or camu camu), mesquite powder, and cacao nibs around to make protein bars. Having finger food around is especially important at the beginning. If you can't find these in your local health food store look online.

Amla and camu camu might sound like insignificant ingredients, but they are actually just as important as salt in making protein bar and breakfast cereal recipes. Adding these sources of vitamin C goes a long way in giving these recipes flavor while increasing their digestibility so that they do not lay heavy in your stomach. Cereals are a staple in our diet. This no accident. Cereal recipes in this book combine vitamins A, C, and E so that your body gets what it came for when it craves cereal.

Buy powders such as fo-ti, carob, mesquite, maca, lucuma, shan zhu yu and shan yao. They are all earthy flavors that we could all grow to like and powders that can serve as alternatives to coffee, red wine, and chocolate. Find them at your local health food store or online. Try them all. It's important to have alternatives and a variety.

Purchase greens on a weekly basis so that you always have a salad ready to go. A salad can be the base for lunch, dinner, or a light snack. You can add fish, beef, chicken, or eggs (so stock up on these, too) to any salad, and you have a meal. Or you can go without animal products and make the salad a quick, light snack that never has to go in the oven. The trick to salad is that you need all the flavors that satisfy your palate. A winter salad begins with chopped kale, collards, and/or green chard, while a summer salad begins with salad greens. Summer salads can continue with berries, cheese, broccoli, sprouts and other fruit. In the summer, you can add almond, walnut, or sesame oil as these flavors taste great with berries and fruit. A winter salad calls for cranberries, cruciferous vegetables, and nuts. Then, use unrefined olive oil and lemon. Salads for any seasons can have any combination of the following: peas, radishes, dates, beets, carrots, hearts of palm, chopped tomatoes, and herbs like dill, parsley, basil, thyme, and mint. These combinations of flavors are always very satisfying.

Keep zucchini around and buy yourself a spiralizer (can be found on Amazon for under $30). Hot marinara sauce over spiralized zucchini with grated Pecorino Romano is an easy meal. We all keep tomato sauce or canned tomatoes and pasta around. Make it a habit to reach for spiralized zucchini instead. Just this small change removes a common food allergen (grains) and deposits enzymes, chlorophyll, and fiber into our diet. Drizzle unrefined olive oil and season spiralized zucchini with salt and pepper as you would your pasta.

Have unrefined walnut oil and pomegranate or cherry concentrate around to make seasonal spiced fruit. I add oils to recipes on a regular basis. Look for fresh unrefined oils online and keep them in your refrigerator. I believe oils by Flora and Now to be fresh.

If you are a salt lover, you can indulge in hiziki, wakame, or arame. These sea vegetables can be purchased online and seasoned with raw tahini and Mrs. Bragg's Liquid Aminos. Sea vegetables are salty, and a sea vegetable salad can really hit the spot when you squeeze half an orange, add chopped cilantro, and a hard pear. Mrs. Bragg's is a great alternative to soy sauce. Keep some in your pantry and use it for any recipe that calls for soy sauce, as soy sauce contains gluten and yeast.

An important investment is a high-powered blender. You don't really even need a juicer unless you are an athlete or have an illness and need a concentrated influx of nutrients. Otherwise, juice just gives you an insulin spike because the juice comes without the necessary fiber required to mediate absorption. A high-powered blender can make you a green juice. Blend a glass of filtered water, a few green chard or collard green leaves, ½ apple, and a carrot. The fiber in your juice is a plus. Dehydrators aren't a good investment either. Eating dehydrated foods isn't recommended for optimal health. Making nut mylk, seed mylk, nut cheese, and vegan fruit pudding may or may not be possible in your regular blender or with a bullet. If you find it's not creamy enough, you should increase the horsepower of your blender. Two good brands are the Vitamix and Waring blenders.

Please purchase Lugol's Iodine Solution if you do not consume shellfish on a weekly basis, as iodine and trace minerals are noticeably missing from our diet. Put a few drops into your homemade mylks and juices. Fulvic acid is a great source of trace minerals. Add to your juice.

Food-grade hydrogen peroxide is a cleaning product many of us have never heard of. It's as effective as chloride bleach in whitening laundry, bleaching floors, and killing bacteria in our kitchens and bathrooms. It kills bacteria and parasites in raw vegetables and sprouts while being nontoxic. Chlorine is especially damaging to our thyroid, and you would be surprised how often we are exposed to it. Chlorine is in our pools and in our drinking water. Bleach, which contains chlorine, has effectively replaced food-grade hydrogen peroxide. Chlorine is used to wash shrimp. When making sprouts or soaking seeds and nuts, which should be common practice in your kitchen, food-grade hydrogen peroxide kills mold and bacteria. Putting a drop into your water in the morning adds oxygen to your body and is very beneficial for good health. Store it in a cool place. Be careful when handling, as food-grade hydrogen peroxide is often very concentrated and can burn.

Making these additions to your refrigerator and pantry will ensure that your experiences with this book and changing your diet are good ones.

RECITE TABLE OF CONTENTS

A Note on Raw Foods:

A raw foods diet is not intended as a long-term regimen. Complete raw foods diets should only run from about 1-2 weeks. Consuming raw or undercooked meats, poultry, seafood, shellfish, or eggs may increase your risk of foodborne illness, especially if you have a medical condition. Consult your nutritionist or physician for advice on undergoing a raw foods diet.

These recipes are very interchangeable, so I have combined them into one section.

In the Morning: Beverages and More

Getting off to a good start in the morning is imperative. We awaken in a dehydrated state, so drinking three glasses of filtered water is the best practice. I also used to do at least forty-five minutes of intense exercise on a stationary bike immediately after the water to help keep my hyperactivity down in the morning. Make sure you enter into a state of deep, rhythmic breathing. This will ground you immediately. Set your machine to an incline if need be to stress your muscles, as opposed to peddling furiously.

Coffee and hot chocolate are the drinks of choice in the morning. These stimulants are also food allergens. Since having cravings for caffeine, found in both coffee and chocolate, may come as a result of being low on free-form amino acids, these recipes will focus on free-form amino acids.

Having a warm alternative is nice. Coffea is a hot drink in the morning loaded with antioxidants and nutrients that keep you calm and receptive. This is my coffee drink since the caffeine found in coffee makes me uptight and decaffeinated coffee is full of chemicals. There is a naturally decaffeinated coffee from the gut of elephants that is extremely expensive, which caused me to lose interest entirely.

Coffea Drink

- 1½ cups hot water or goat's milk
- 1 tsp fresh herbs: He Shou Wu, Shan Yao, or Shan Zhu Yu (or any combination of those)
- Pinch of cinnamon
- 1 tsp raw honey

✓ Blend ingredients for 11 seconds or until desired consistency is reached; serve immediately.

Note: The coffea in the photo above contains a handful of soaked almonds. Nuts need to be soaked for 8 hours. For easy access, I recommend always keeping a cup of nuts that have been previously soaked in the fridge. That said, this recipe is good with or without the nuts.

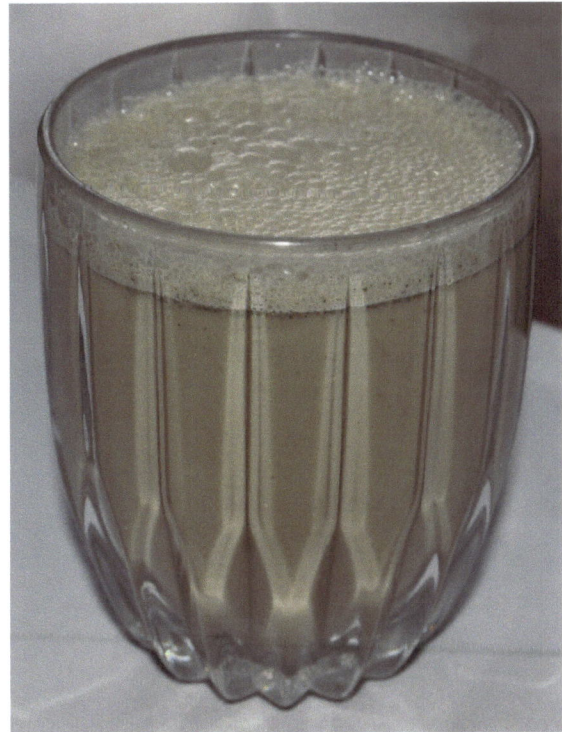

Green Shot

This recipe is recommended by Dr. Gerson, author of numerous books including *The Beautiful Truth, A Cancer Therapy: Results of Fifty Cases,* and *The Cure of Advanced Cancer* and the documentary *Dying to Have Known.*

During his life, Dr. Gerson believed that cancer and other ailments came as a result of poor oxygen and nutrition in the body. He prescribed 13 glasses of carrot, apple, green chard juice with supplements daily to patients, and many got better. His findings were so amazing that to this day people follow his program. To learn more, purchase his book *Gerson Therapy* or watch *Dying to Have Known* by the Gerson Institute.

Dr. Gerson contended that the nutrients in juiced green leaves are lost within 30 minutes. As such, drink green juice quickly. Green supplements made from marine phytoplankton or a sea green, such as crushed chlorella, spirulina, and blue green algae, can also be added to your diet easily. Please remember that the most nutritious juice drinks are unpasteurized.

- ♦ 3 large green chard leaves
- ♦ 1 large carrot
- ♦ 1 apple

- ✓ Using a Norwalk juicer or a high-powered blender, press above ingredients and serve immediately.

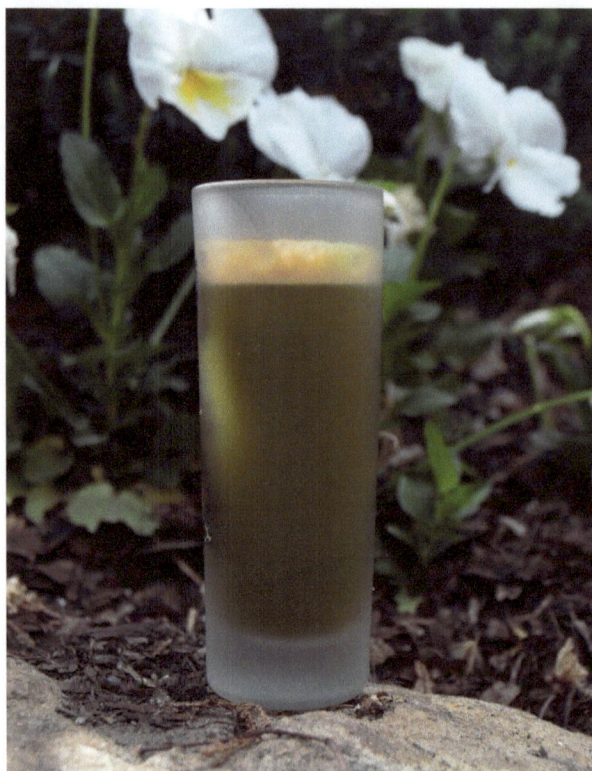

Mocha Protein Shake

When we think of protein shakes, we immediately think of chocolate or whey. The truth is there are other equally nourishing powders that tasty, nourishing shakes can be created with. Maca, mesquite, shan zhu yu, shan yao, fo-ti (aka he shou wu), carob, and lucuma are a few excellent flavors to play around with.

Maca Smoothie

- ½ tsp maca
- 1 Tbsp mesquite
- 1½ cups water (hot or cold)
- 1 organic banana with peel*
- Handful of soaked macadamia nuts
- 1 tsp sea salt
- ✓ Blend ingredients for 11 seconds or until desired consistency is reached; serve immediately.

The banana peel is optional. You can't taste it. It adds fiber and who knows what other nutrients and helps with hemorrhoids, as per Henry C. Lu, author of Chinese System of Food Cures, *who explains that bananas with peels have an upward-moving energy.*

Mocha Smoothie

- 1 tsp Shan Yao
- 1 tsp Shan Zhu Yu
- 1½ cups water (hot or cold)
- Dash of cinnamon
- 1 tsp local honey
- 1 Tbsp colostrum or goat milk powder
- 1 tsp sea salt

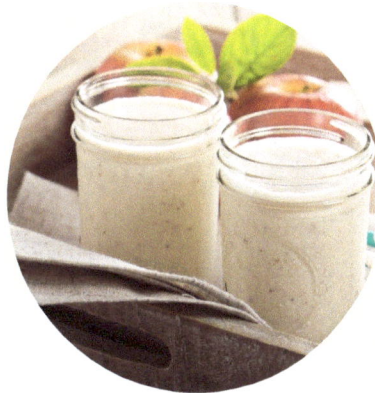

- ✓ Blend ingredients for 11 seconds or until desired consistency is reached; serve immediately.

Carob Drink

+ 1 Tbsp carob
+ 1 Tbsp sunflower, almond, hazelnut, or raw tahini butter
+ 1 Tbsp local honey or royal jelly
+ 1 cup water (hot or cold)
+ Small piece of Aloe vera

✓ Blend ingredients for 11 seconds or until desired consistency is reached; serve immediately.

Mint Smoothie

+ 1 cup mint leaves or drops of essential oil of mint (not peppermint)
+ ½ avocado
+ 1 Tbsp lucuma powder/ honey/royal jelly
+ 2 ½ cups rice mylk or nut mylk
+ 1-2 tablets of chlorella, spirulina, or blue green algae
+ ¼ tsp sea salt

✓ Blend ingredients for 11 seconds or until desired consistency is reached; serve immediately.

Rich Dessert Smoothie

- ♦ ½ avocado
- ♦ 2 tsp honey/royal jelly
- ♦ 2½ cups rice mylk
- ♦ ¼ tsp sea salt

- ✓ Blend ingredients for 11 seconds or until desired consistency is reached; serve immediately.

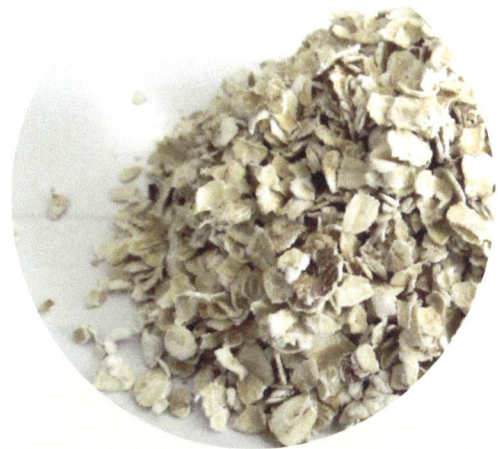

Protein Smoothie

- ♦ 1 ripe plantain
- ♦ 1 cup goat milk
- ♦ ¼ cup oat lakes
- ♦ 1-2 drops sea minerals/fulvic acid
- ♦ 1 tsp sea salt

- ✓ Blend ingredients for 11 seconds or until desired consistency is reached; serve immediately.

Quinoa Smoothie

- ½ cup cooked amaranth or quinoa
- 1 cup goat milk, rice mylk, or seed mylk
- 1-3 pitted dates or 1 Tbsp local raw honey
- 1 tsp sea salt

- ✓ Boil amaranth or quinoa in 1½ cups water for 30 minutes or until soft and then blend with other ingredients for 11 seconds or until desired consistency is reached. Serve immediately hot or with ice for a cold drink.

These are my hot chocolates since my ADHD acts up when I overdo cacao.

Mocha Shake on Steroids

By adding supplements to your favorite smoothie recipe above, you can increase their nutritional value even more:

- ✓ Add cranberry, cherry, blueberry or pomegranate concentrate for added antioxidants.
- ✓ Add camu camu or amla powder, which are antioxidants in the form of vitamin C.
- ✓ Use freshly-peeled aloe vera, which contains free-form amino acids as well as dries up the excess mucus created in our bodies by the overconsumption of cow dairy.
- ✓ You can also add chlorella, spirulina, and blue green algae to remove heavy metals from the body and deposit chlorophyll, which oxygenates the blood. Too much chlorella for a prolonged period of time can cause cravings for bread and cookies, so don't overdo it.
- ✓ Soaked chia seeds hydrate our bodies and are full of B vitamins, protein and fiber.
- ✓ Ground eggshells (boil to kill bacteria) add bioavailable calcium to your diet.

Easy Rich & Creamy Dessert

- ½ ripe avocado
- 2 Tbsp almond oil
- ½ cup lucuma powder
- ¼ tsp grated ginger
- Dash of salt
- Minced pineapple

✓ Puree ingredients in a food processor and serve with minced pineapple.

Optional Recipe to Above

- One avocado
- 2 Tbsp carob
- 2 Tbsp raw tahini
- Your choice of healthy sweetener to taste (raw agave, yacon syrup, or raw honey)
- 1 tsp orange rind, grated
- Dash of salt

✓ Puree ingredients in a food processor and serve.

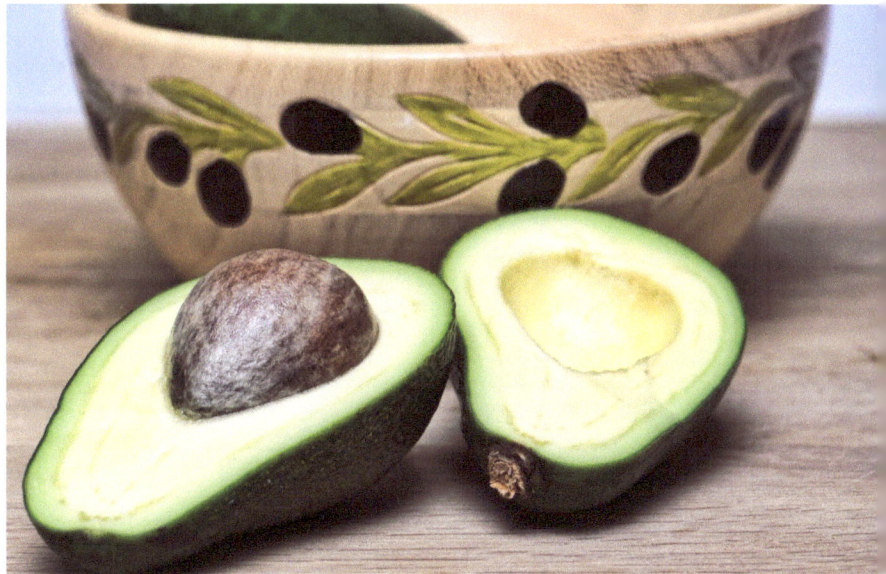

Vegan Mylks

There is so much talk about CoQ10, which aids in the production of cellular energy and is found abundantly in our kidneys, liver, and heart. Statin drugs prescribed to lower cholesterol have come under fire for blocking this vital energy enzyme in the body, often leading to heart malfunction. Sprouted seeds are an abundant source of CoQ10 and are a good source of healthy fats and minerals such as magnesium, calcium, and zinc. Seeds make great mylks.

Most nuts also make a delicious mylk, so experiment with soaked macadamia, pecans, hazelnuts, and almonds nuts and add vanilla flavor, cloves, cinnamon, nutmeg, and allspice for additional flavor. If the fibers bother you, pour the mylk through cheesecloth to remove them. Please remember to keep nuts that have been previously soaked in your refrigerator at all times. Refer to the area entitled "grocery list" for nut soaking instructions.

Pumpkin Seed Mylk

One hour before, soak shelled pumpkin seeds (pepitas) in filtered water, and then discard water. Pumpkin seeds are known to have anti-inflammatory properties for arthritis, be beneficial for prostate health, and have cholesterol-lowering qualities. They are high in zinc, which helps to regulate blood sugar levels (imperative for mental clarity). Pumpkin Seeds are also an anti-parasitic and high in potassium, which protects our bones against salt in processed foods. Add seeds to your everyday diet.

- ¾ cup pepitas
- 5 cups filtered water
- 1 coin ginger
- ¼ cup local raw honey
- ¼ tsp sea salt

✓ Blend ingredients for 11 seconds or until desired consistency is reached and serve.

Optional: Replace the sea salt with ¼ tsp of sea minerals or fulvic acid.

Will keep in refrigerator for up to one week

Sesame Seed Mylk

- ¼ cup raw tahini (sesame paste)
- 5 cups filtered water
- ¼ cup local raw honey
- ½ tsp salt
- ½ tsp amla

✓ Blend ingredients for 11 seconds or until desired consistency is reached. Serve.
Optional: Add ¼ tsp of fulvic acid.

Will keep in refrigerator for up to one week

Hemp Seed Mylk

This is a great source of omega 6 for vegetarians.

- ½ cup hemp seeds
- 5 cups filtered water
- ¼ cup local raw honey
- ¼ tsp salt
- ½ tsp amla

✓ Blend ingredients for 11 seconds or until desired consistency is reached. Serve.

Will keep in refrigerator for up to one week

Rice Mylk

- 4 cups water, split
- ½ cup washed brown rice
- ¼ cup raw local honey
- ½ tsp fulvic acid
- ¼ tsp salt

✓ Boil 2 cups of water. Then, add ½ cup washed brown rice. Boil again and cover. Simmer for 40 minutes.

✓ Pour water/rice mixture into blender and add 2 cups water. Add remaining ingredients and blend for 11 seconds or until desired consistency is reached.

✓ Pour through cheesecloth; allow to sit for 30 minutes until fully drained.

Will keep in refrigerator for up to one week

Optional ingredients that may be added to any of the above mylk recipes:

- 1 Tbsp eggshell
- 1 Tbsp pearl
- 1 Tbsp goat milk powder and/or colostrum
- 2 drops of Lugol's Iodine Solution
- 1 drop of fulvic acid

Sheep and goat milk are easily digested and can be added to your nut mylk as a source of B-12. Note: B-12 is not found within a vegan diet.

You can also play with fruit pulps in the summer, which are widely available at Latin markets. They open up a whole new world of flavors, if the same old flavors have you down. Flavors like sour sop, passion fruit, blackberry, Tree Lulu and tree tomatoes have many anti-cancer and blood-pressure-lowering properties. Add these pulps to water or your favorite nut mylk with brown sugar and a dash of salt.

Warm Winter Breakfast

Eating seasonally helps keep our bodies in balance. Many of us begin our day with fruit. In the winter, beginning our day with squash is the equivalent since squash and root vegetables are Mother Earth's winter fruit. Complex carbohydrates are also a healing way to begin our day when compared to breakfast foods such as eggs, bacon, toast, hot coco, sugary cereals, and pasteurized juice, which require lots of insulin to digest and throw our bodies out of balance, as I mentioned. Eating in this way sends the brain on an emotional roller coaster if we don't burn it off during a strenuous activity.

Winter Squash

- 1 acorn or butternut squash
- 1 cup pomegranate seeds or cranberries
- ¼ cup unrefined almond/walnut/butter/sesame oil
- 1 tsp of your choice of cloves, cinnamon, nutmeg, mace, or allspice
- 1 apple

✓ Rinse butternut or acorn squash and slice in half. Scoop seeds into a separate dish.
✓ Bake seeds at 200°F until crisp, about 15 minutes. Place squash halves in a separate dish face down and bake at 325°F until soft, about 30 minutes.

Serve with additional pomegranate seeds or any of the following:

Toasted seeds

Handful of blanched cranberries

Unrefined oil of your choosing (butter oil, walnut, sesame, or almond oil)

Dash of any combination of cloves, cinnamon, nutmeg, mace, or allspice

Crunchy apple, cut in large, bite-sized cubes

The apple is a nice touch for flavor and for texture. Your teeth naturally want to chew, and the large pieces of apple give you that opportunity.

Warm Breakfast Porridge

Porridges are a wonderful way to begin your day since they tend to be very balancing, lower cholesterol, and are full of B vitamins. B vitamins are brain food.

- ½ cup plantain flour
- 2 cups water or goat's or coconut milk
- ¼ tsp ginger, grated
- ¼ tsp green chili, minced
- 1 Tbsp brown sugar
- 1 tsp sea salt
- 1 Tbsp coconut or walnut oil
- ¼ cup cherries

- ✓ Dilute ½ cup plantain flour in ½ cup of cold water and add to 2 cups boiling water (or goat or coconut milk).
- ✓ Boil for 15 minutes, stirring constantly. Remove from heat. Add ¼ tsp of grated ginger, pinch of minced green chili, and 1 Tbsp brown sugar. Add a dash of sea salt and 1 tsp of coconut oil. Serve warm over cherries.

Porridge Cereal Template

Grains and greens go together, so take a shot of green juice with this. Please refer to my Green Shot recipe, or if you feel lazy, crush a spirulina or chlorella tablet and stir into fresh pressed carrot/apple juice.

- 2 cups rice mylk (or almond, goat, or coconut milk)
- ¼ cup your favorite non-glutinous grain (quinoa, sorghum, teff, amaranth, millet, or oat)
- Raw local honey, cinnamon, allspice, nutmeg, and/or salt to taste

- ✓ Heat mylk until simmering. Add grain (remember to wash grains in sieve before cooking). Simmer, stirring constantly for 30 minutes or until grain is soft. Season to taste with any or all of the above.
- ✓ Serve alongside a fruit of your choice. Adding a tablespoon of your favorite oil makes this rich as well as nourishing. In the summer, choose coconut oil, as medium-chain triglycerides feed the brain directly. In the winter, try unrefined almond, walnut, sesame, or hazelnut oil. Flora and Now oils have many flavors to choose from, and their oils are unrefined.

Breakfast Sandwich

Per serving:
- 1 apple, sliced
- Portion of sliced avocado
- Collard green leaf, deveined
- Salt to taste
- Olive oil

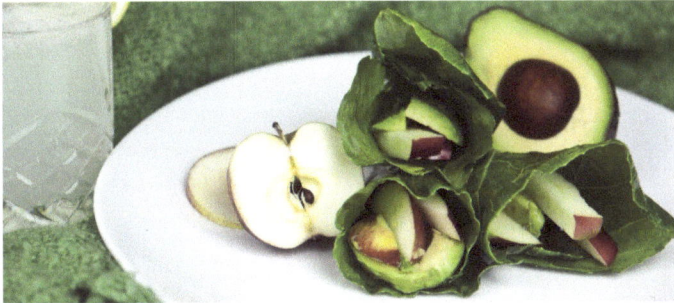

✓ Rub a sliced apple and avocado and collard green leaf (vein removed) with salt and unrefined olive oil. Wrap apple and avocado in leaf.

In the summer, you can serve with nut mylk.

Breakfast Cereals

The reason cereals are a life-sustaining food is that they contain the nutrition combination of vitamins A, C, and E. When taken together, these nutrients have a synergistic nutritional benefit to the body that requires little insulin to digest. Sprouted seeds, salt, and sweet and tart fruit provide all the nutrients and flavors present in boxed cereal plus many more, all in a way that is more bioavailable. Try these cereal combinations. If you experience cravings, try amino acid therapy, urine therapy, or a parasite purge program.

Sunflower Seed Breakfast Cereal

Soak seeds for one hour.

- ◆ 1 tsp poppy seeds or black sesame seeds, soaked
- ◆ ¼ cup raw sunflower seeds, hulled and soaked
- ◆ 1 cup nut mylk or 1 cup water with 1 Tbsp walnut oil
- ◆ 1 chopped apple
- ◆ 2 dates, pitted
- ◆ 1 tsp sea salt
- ◆ Handful fresh berries, kiwi (peeled), or other tart fruit

Sprinkle with camu camu or amla for extra vitamin C

✓ Soak nuts. Place ingredients in a bowl and cover with nut mylk or water/oil combination.

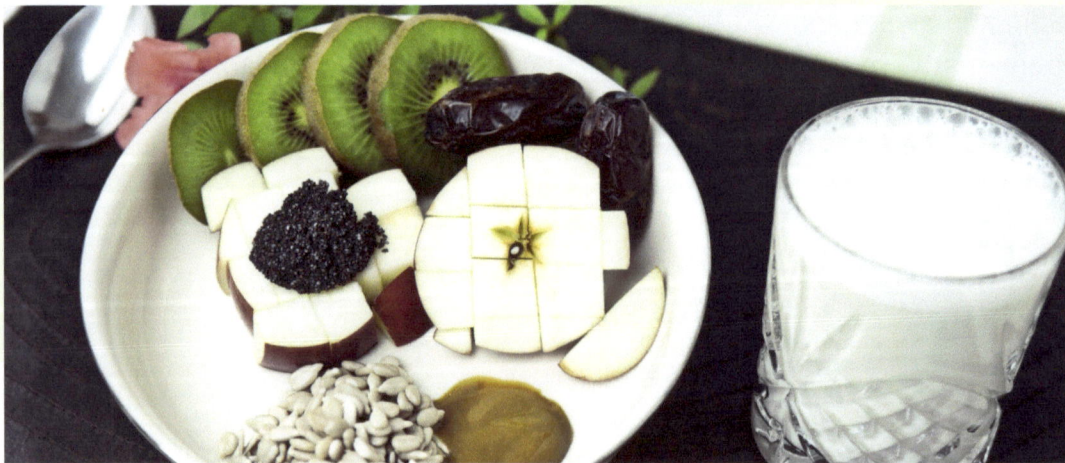

Chia Seed Cereal

- 1 Tbsp chia seeds
- ¾ cup filtered water
- 1 Tbsp goat milk powder or colostrum powder
- 1 Tbsp local honey
- ¼ cup berries

✓ Combine chia seeds and water in a glass and allow to absorb the water for about 15 minutes. Stir in milk powder, and top with honey and berries.

Sprouted Breakfast Cereal

Refer to the sprouting section for information and directions (see page 86).

- 2 Tbsp buckwheat, sprouted and whole oat groats
- 1 cup nut mylk or 1 cup water with 1 Tbsp walnut oil
- 1 apple, chopped
- Handful fresh berries
- Sprinkle of camu camu
- 2-3 pitted dates or 1 Tbsp local honey

✓ Place ingredients in a bowl and cover with nut mylk or water/oil combination.

Optional cereal ingredients include the following:

Raw cacao nibs, oat flakes, sprouted whole buckwheat groats, sprouted whole oat groats, royal jelly/bee pollen, lucuma rings, local seasonal fruit, yacon syrup, raw coconut nectar, and agave.

You can add your favorite cereal if you like as well.

Plantain Breakfast

How often do we take a banana and go? Plantains have more protein and less sugar, making plantains a better choice for a quick snack on the run. A ripe plantain and mocha shake can really hit the spot. The Mocha Smoothie is depicted here to give you food combination ideas. I find these smoothies give me a strong sense of well-being and reduce my cravings for coffee, hot chocolate, and red wine—which I crave on a consistent basis.

- ♦ 1 plantain, baked or raw
- ♦ 1-2 Tbsp butter oil or cube of cheese

- ✓ Bake plantain with peel in conventional oven for 20-30 minutes at 300°F or peel a raw plantain and serve. Pour butter oil over plantain. Optional sides include cheese, spiced season fruit, mylk, and coffea drink.

Nut Cheese

Eight to ten hours before, soak 2 cup sof nuts.

Options include almonds, hazelnuts, pecans, macadamia or pine nuts.

Note: Cashews and pistachios are missing from this list, as they do not digest well. Peanuts are a bean, not a nut, and cannot be eaten raw. This is not to bash peanuts because all foods have one negative quality or another, but peanuts are particularly high in aflatoxin, a carcinogenic mold. For that reason, I use them very sparingly.

- ♦ 2 cups Marcona almonds, soaked
- ♦ ⅓ cup filtered water
- ♦ ½ tsp honey, yacon syrup, raw agave, or coconut nectar
- ♦ 1 tsp sea salt

✓ Soak nuts. Combine above ingredients in a blender. Blend for 11 seconds at a time until smooth. Allow mixture to cool in between blending for a minute or so.

✓ Stop here when making cream. If you need more water to puree, you can wrap the mixture in cheesecloth and allow it to drain overnight

To make soft cheese, you need some kick, so add any of the following:

♦ ¼ tsp mustard seed, ground, or mustard seed oil
♦ ¼ tsp fennel seeds or ground dill seeds
♦ ¼ tsp raw vinegar
♦ ¼ tsp miso
♦ 1 garlic tooth, creamed
♦ 1 dash salt
♦ Olive oil

✓ Smash garlic tooth using flat of knife and allow to sit with dash of salt and a spot of olive oil for 5 minutes. Blend all ingredients with the Nut Cheese mixture.

✓ Soak nuts in plenty of filtered water with a few drops of food-grade hydrogen peroxide to kill mold and bacteria. Some like to strain this nut cheese mixture in cheesecloth and allow it to ferment in order to make a harder cheese, but I've always been satisfied with a soft cheese, and the miso does a great job of giving nuts a cheese-like flavor.

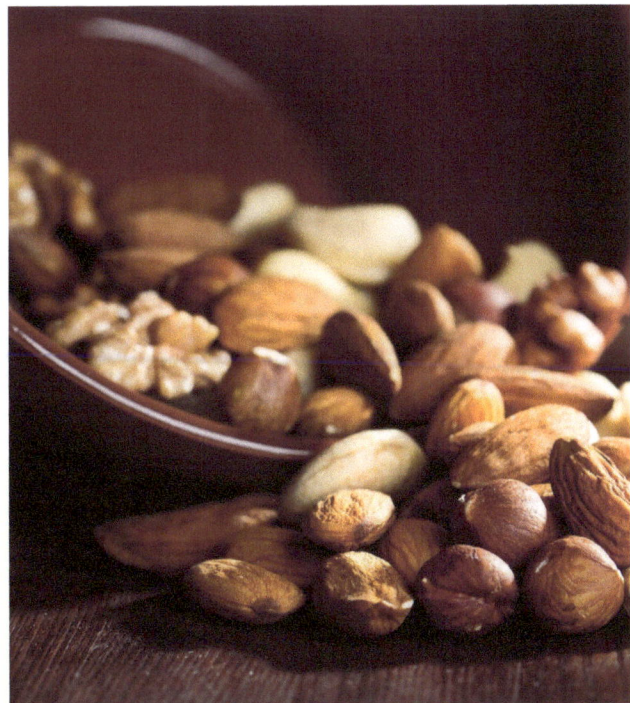

Versatile Vegan Mousse

Twenty-four hours prior, soak 2 Tbsp wild Irish moss

Eight hours prior, soak 1 cup raw macadamia or almonds

- 1 cup Marcona almonds, soaked, or macadamia nuts, soaked
- 2 Tbsp wild Irish moss
- 1 cup young coconut meat
- ½ cup pitted dates
- ½ cup raw honey
- 1 Tbsp water
- Few drops of fulvic acid or other sea mineral
- ½ cup your choice of fruit pulp

✓ Blend above ingredients 11 seconds at a time until smooth, allowing mixture to cool in between blending activity. Once smooth, blend with fruit pulp of your choice. (Flavors I've seen in the frozen section of Latin grocers include blackberry, passion fruit, sour sop, and guava.) Pour into mold and allow to set in the refrigerator for 5 hours.

Option to above:

Coconut meat, dates, macadamia or almond nuts and wild Irish moss are a great base for any pie. You can basically flavor this any way you want. For added color and flavor, experiment with a swirl.

Swirl ideas:

You can make chocolate swirl, pomegranate concentrate swirl, cranberry swirl, passion fruit swirl, mango/orange, kiwi/lime, peach/ripe pear, mandarin/tangerine/orange, or any combination you fancy. You can do orange/sweet potato in the winter to somewhat follow the seasons, though coconut is for the summer.

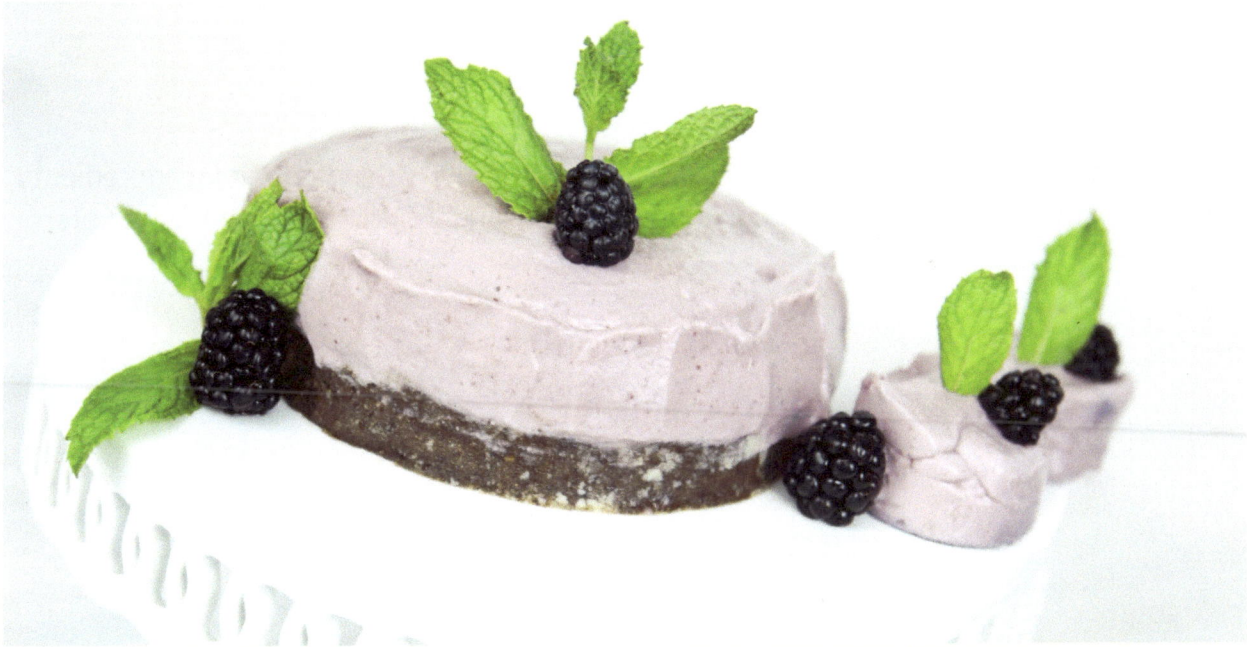

Coconut Mousse Swirl

- 1 Tbsp raw cacao powder
- ¼ cup coconut nectar or raw yacon syrup
- Pinch of salt
- 1 orange, mango, or kiwi, peeled
- ¼ cup honey
- Salt to taste

✓ Combine first three ingredients in dish using a spoon. Blend remaining ingredients until they reach the desired consistency and swirl into mixture from the first step using a small spoon.

SPROUTING

Sprouting in order to supplement your diet

Sprouts contain massive quantities of every nutrient present in the whole bean/vegetable/grain that we eat. All sprouts are mineral-rich and nutrient-dense foods. Sprouts add free-form amino acids and enzymes to any meal. As you know, free-form

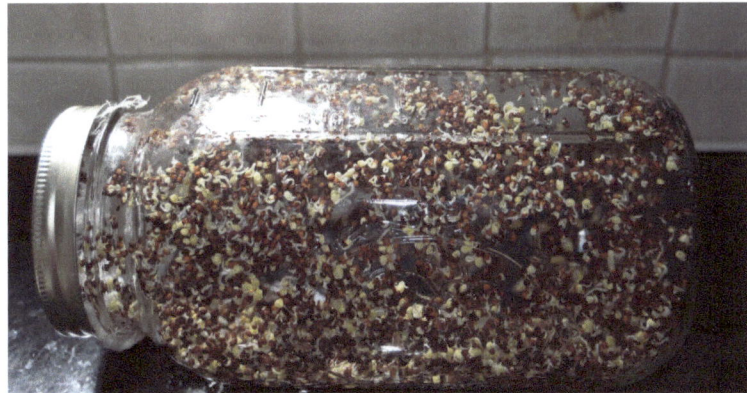

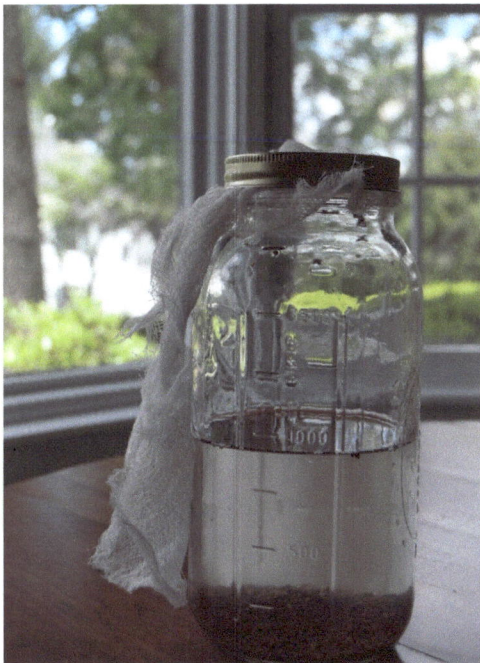

amino acids are the raw materials that our bodies create our feel-good hormones from, without which we can easily have cravings for sugar, nicotine, aspartame, and other drugs. Getting extra nutrition from sprouts is best because, bite for bite, they contain many times the nutritional value of mature vegetables. Sprouts contain nutrients that are highly bioavailable. Their live enzymes make them more bioavailable than chalky vitamins made in a lab or even those found in cooked foods. Those enzymes reduce the burden imposed on cells during the digestive process. The fiber in sprouts is an added benefit; and finally, they add texture and flavor to our salads, sandwiches, and soups.

What to sprout

You can sprout whatever you like and in the quantities you like. That said, I realize we all have other things to juggle in our lives. I recommend you only sprout what you know you can incorporate into your diet, so if you like grains sprout whole buckwheat and oat groats once or twice a month. Those who prefer beans should sprout lentils and mung beans on a monthly basis. Broccoli seeds are my favorite sprouts because they offer the most nutritional value of any vegetable. They are loaded with antioxidants such as sulforaphane, which protect us from the damaging effects of free radicals and are effective in preventing many types of cancer. Broccoli and other cruciferous sprouts also contain large amounts of plant compounds that balance our hormones, such as diindolylmethane (DIM), which has a balancing effect on the hormones estrogen and testosterone. These healthy plant compounds help our bodies break down estrogen into healthy versions for improvements in bodybuilding, sexual health, and healthy aging. To learn more, read about DIM online. Enzymes found in raw foods reduce the burden imposed on cells during the digestive process.

What to start with:

- 1 half-gallon-sized Mason jar
- 6 square-inches of cheese cloth
- 1 lid
- 1 tsp food-grade hydrogen peroxide
- ¼ cup broccoli seeds or 1 cup buckwheat or whole oat groats or 1 cup lentils/mung beans

✓ Place 4-6 cups of filtered water in your Mason jar with 1 tsp food-grade hydrogen peroxide and whatever it is you are sprouting, whether it's grain, beans, or seeds. Cover with cheesecloth, secure with lid, and allow to stand for 8-10 hours or overnight.

✓ The next morning, drain jar, add fresh water, drain jar again, and add fresh water. Drain and lay the jar on its side for 8-12 hours.

✓ Repeat step 2 until your grain/beans/seeds have tiny roots, about 1½ days.

✓ Once you see roots, rinse contents through a sieve and place on an open tray to dry. Cover with sieve to protect from flies or other insects. Once dry, place sprouts in a container and refrigerate. The shelf life is one week when refrigerated.

Raw Sprinkles and Crusts

Raw Sprinkles (for buckwheat or oat grouts)

I make this regularly and keep it handy as a dessert topping or for cereal. Please refer to my spicy seasonal fruit recipe for an easy dessert combination, which you may add seasoned grain sprouts to.

Prepare, sprout, and dry grouts two days in advance.

- ♦ ¼ cup whole buckwheat or oat grouts
- ♦ Coconut nectar or raw honey, mace, allspice, cloves, cinnamon, nutmeg, and salt

- ✓ Sprout and dry whole buckwheat or oat groats. Once grain is dry, you may season and save in Tupperware in fridge for up to a week. Add seasonings of your choice to the dried sprouts.

Crusts

Seed and grain crusts make a wonderful base or crunchy topping that you can use in a dessert or a breakfast treat. Sprouted buckwheat and oat groats contain all amino acids needed by the body as well as the fiber, calcium, minerals, enzymes, and CoQ10 for optimal brain function. These crust alternatives allow you to avoid gluten and processed crusts that contain food allergens.

Easy Crust

- ◆ 1 cup almond flour*
- ◆ ½ cup dates
- ◆ Sea salt, cinnamon, nutmeg, cloves to taste

✓ Add ingredients to a food processor and pulse until well ground and fluffy. The pliable mixture, when packed, becomes a crust for your favorite pie.

To make your own sprouted almond flour, purchase raw almonds directly from a farm. (I like Snack Farms.) Soak almonds for 8 hours. Discard any nuts that float. Allow to dry and then grind in coffee grinder.

Sprouted Grain Crust

Two days before, sprout whole oat groats and buckwheat groats using the sprouting instructions provided.

Once the grains have been sprouted and have air-dried, grind them in a coffee grinder to obtain sprouted gluten-free grain flour.

- ◆ 1 cup sprouted gluten-free grain flour
- ◆ ½ cup dates
- ◆ ¼ tsp amla powder or 1 Tbsp freshly squeezed lemon juice
- ◆ 1 Tbsp brown sugar
- ◆ ½ Tbsp walnut oil
- ◆ Sea salt, cinnamon, cloves to taste

✓ Add ingredients to a food processor and pulse until well ground and fluffy. The pliable mixture, when packed, becomes a crust for your favorite pie.

Seed Crust

- 1 cup flaxseeds
- 2 Tbsp coffee
- ½ cup pitted dates
- ¼ tsp amla powder or 1 Tbsp freshly squeezed lemon juice
- Pinch of salt, cinnamon, nutmeg, mace, and allspice

✓ Add flaxseeds and coffee to a coffee grinder or food processor and pulse. Add remaining ingredients until well ground and fluffy. The pliable mixture, when packed, becomes a crust for your favorite pie.

Sesame Date Crust

- 1 cup sesame or chia seeds
- ½ cup pitted dates
- ¼ tsp amla powder or 1 Tbsp freshly squeezed lemon juice
- Pinch of salt, cinnamon, nutmeg, mace, and allspice to taste

✓ Add seeds to a coffee grinder or food processor and pulse. Add remaining ingredients and pulse until well ground and fluffy. Pliable mixture when packed becomes a crust for your favorite pie.

Nut Crust

Soak your favorite nut for 8 hours and allow to dry for 8 hours.

- ◆ 1 cup sprouted nut flour*
- ◆ ½ cup pitted dates
- ◆ ¼ tsp amla powder or 1 Tbsp freshly squeezed lemon juice
- ◆ ¼ tsp salt, ¼ tsp cinnamon, ¼ tsp nutmeg, and pinch of cloves to taste.

✓ Grind nuts in coffee grinder to create sprouted nut flour. Add flour to food processor and add remaining ingredients. Pulse until well ground and fluffy. The pliable mixture, when packed, becomes a crust for your favorite pie.

*To make your own sprouted nut flour, purchase raw nuts. Soak for 8 hours. Allow to dry and then grind in coffee grinder.

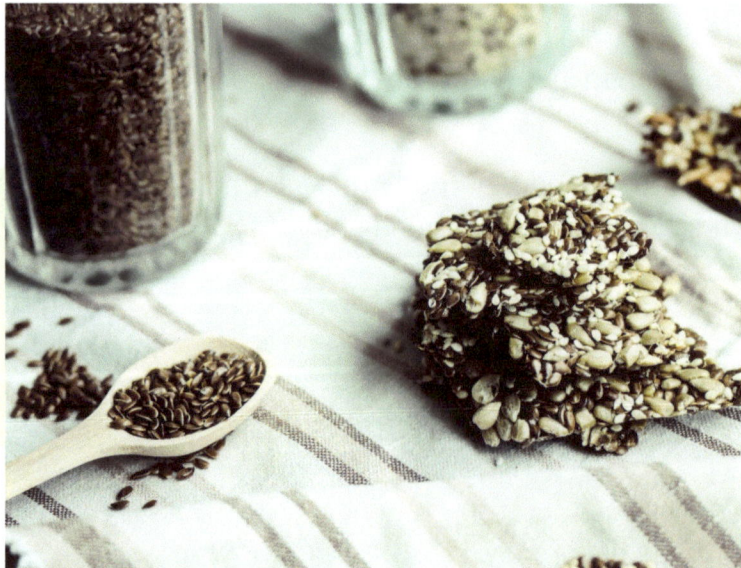

Fruits, Syrups, and Desserts

Seasonal Spiced Fruits

Berry syrups can turn any chopped fruit, wild yam, butternut or acorn squash into a tasty dessert because they contain the flavors your tongue wants to taste in a dessert.

Berry concentrates contain powerful antioxidants that burn fat, are very nourishing for the endocrine system, and remove toxins at a cellular level. Cherry concentrate is high in melatonin, which regulates sleep cycle; and pomegranate and raspberry concentrates help with the production of progesterone in the body, which assists in removing belly fat, building bone, repairing damaged nerves in the brain, and contains nourishing heart fats. Phycocyanin, found in blueberries and spirulina, have anti-inflammatory effects and evacuate toxins at a cellular level, all giving us more energy!

Pomegranate Syrup

Eight hours prior, soak nuts.

- ¼ cup pomegranate concentrate
- ¼ cup walnut, almond, or macadamia nut oil
- ¼ cup raw local honey, coconut nectar, or yacon syrup
- ¼ cup walnuts, hazelnuts, or pecans, soaked

✓ Combine ingredients in a bowl using a spoon. Pour over fruit or store in your refrigerator for up to a week.*

*The concentrate, oil, and sweetener will keep for a month. It is the soaked nuts that have a shelf life of a week.

This recipe works well with ANY concentrate. Some ideas include:

- ¼ cup cherry concentrate
- ¼ cup raspberry concentrate
- ¼ cup blueberry concentrate
- ¼ cup juice of an orange with a twist of lime

Raw Apple Pie

- 3 apples, peeled, cored, and segmented
- 1 cup cranberries, blanched,* or pomegranate seeds
- 1 cup plums or pitted dates, chopped
- ⅓ cup of your favorite berry sauce recipe above
- ¼ cup cacao nibs
- 1 tsp amla or camu camu powder
- ¼ tsp sea salt or salt to taste

Optional: 1 Tbsp bee pollen, mulberries, or goji berries

✓ Combine ingredients and serve mixture atop your choice of crust recipes provided earlier.

Optional: Insert raw goat brie or goat ricotta in between crust and fruit. To make other fruit pies, substitute peaches and/or pears for apple. This also makes a great breakfast.

*Easy blanching method: Bring 2 cups of water to boil. Place cranberries in pot for one minute and remove cranberries. Your cranberries are blanched.

Brownies

Brownie recipes make a high-protein chunk great for energy at sporting events. You may add royal jelly, goji berries, mulberries, spirulina/chlorella, cayenne pepper, or any healthy supplement to your brownies.

Mesquite Brownie

One day before, soak pecans/walnuts for 8 hours. Drain and allow to dry on an open plate.

- ½ cup pitted dates
- ⅓ cup nuts, soaked
- ¼ cup raw cacao nibs
- 1 tsp powdered amla or camu camu
- 1 tsp sea salt
- 2 Tbsp mesquite powder

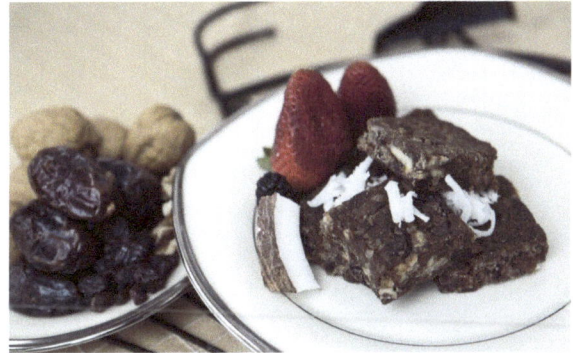

✓ Soak nuts. Combine above ingredients in a food processor. Pulse for 30 seconds at a time until well combined. Place contents on a plate or Tupperware, shape by compressing gently, and allow your protein bar to set. Cut into cubes and serve at room temperature with toasted sunflower seeds or mylk.

Optional: Use toasted sun lower seeds. Take 1 cup raw sun lower seeds in shell. Bake at 275°F for 15 minutes or until the shell is crisp.

Cacao Brownie

Substitute raw cacao powder for the mesquite powder in the recipe above.

Carob Brownie

Substitute raw carob powder for the mesquite powder in the recipe above.

Mocha Brownie

Substitute ¼ cup shan yao & 1 Tbsp shan zhu yu for the mesquite powder in the recipe above. (These herbs taste great together.)

Sweet Coconut Cacao Delight

- ½ cup amaranth
- ½ cup teff grains
- 2½ cups filtered water
- 1 Tbsp coconut nectar or yacon syrup
- 1 Tbsp walnut oil or, during hot weather, coconut oil
- Sea salt to taste

✓ In a covered pot, simmer grain in water with the lid on until soft, stirring occasionally. Remove from stove once grains are soft, about 30 minutes. Add oil, sweetener, and salt to gooey mixture. Place into mold to cool and set. Cut into squares and serve at room temperature.

Optional: Sprinkle with cocoa nibs, mint leaves, and/or berries.

Caramel

This healthy caramel recipe can be added to candied fruit, sprouted grains, soaked nuts, or cheese.

- 1 cup raw coconut nectar, honey, or agave
- 1 Tbsp coconut or walnut oil
- ¼ tsp ground anise seed
- 1 Tbsp water
- ½ tsp sea salt
- ⅛ tsp lemon rind, grated

✓ In a food processor, puree above ingredients.

Grit Snack Squares

- ½ cup grits
- 2 cups water
- 2 Tbsp unrefined coconut oil
- Dash of salt

Optional: Raisins

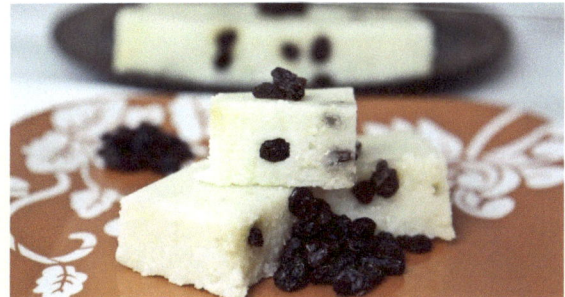

✓ In a covered pot, boil ½ cup grits in water until creamy. Remove from stove, add coconut oil, raisins, and salt.
✓ Place grits in mold to cool and set. Cut into squares and serve at room temperature.

Vegan Ambrosia (three-part recipe)

As we age, we become estrogen-dominant. Walnuts and pomegranates, both in this recipe, create a balance within our bodies and promote balance between estrogen and progesterone. Estrogen dominance is a condition that leads to issues with bone density, sleep patterns, joint pain, vision, energy, and more.

Vegan Sour Cream

One day before, soak Marcona almonds or macadamia nuts for 8 hours.

- 1 cup soaked and peeled nuts
- 1 cup water
- 1 cup young coconut meat
- 1½ Tbsp brown sugar
- 1 Tbsp camu camu or amla powder
- ½ tsp sea salt

Optional: Add 5 drops fulvic acid and 1 drop of Lugol's Iodine Solution.

Fruit

- 2 cups peaches or grapes
- 2 cups mandarins
- 1 cup cherries or berries
- 1 cup hard coconut meat, grated

Berry Syrup

- ¼ cup cherry concentrate or pomegranate concentrate
- ¼ cup raw coconut nectar or raw honey
- ¼ cup sesame/walnut/almond or other unrefined oil by Now or Flora that is liquid at room temperature
- ½ tsp sea salt

Vegan sour cream: Blend ingredients and set aside.

Fruit: In a bowl, combine fruit with grated coconut and set aside.

Berry syrup: In a bowl, stir ingredients together and set aside.

Fold fruit mixture into vegan sour cream. Pour berry syrup over plate; place a scoop of sour cream and fruit mixture on plate and serve chilled or at room temperature.

Keeps in refrigerator for up to one week.

Egg Cream Mixture

Raw, full-fat treats reduce cravings for ice cream. Dr. Weston Price was a prominent dentist in the 1900s whose work revolved around the relationship between nutrition, dental health, and physical health. He wrote about the importance of eating full-fat animal products, such as cage-free eggs, as well as free-range dairy products, meat, and fish for optimal mental clarity and physical health. Dr. Price is also remembered for his work on the synergistic/medicinal qualities associated with combining cod liver fish oil with dairy fat. Many children need extra amounts of animal fat during their developmental years since vitamin B-12 can be difficult to find in the vegan world.

- ¼ cup unhomogenized cream
- 1 egg yolk
- 1 egg white
- 1 tsp vanilla flavor
- ⅛ tsp orange rind
- Pinch of salt

97

✓ Using a hand blender, beat cream for 3 minutes. Add egg yolk and beat for 5 seconds. In a separate bowl, beat egg white until stiff. Fold egg white into egg cream mixture. Add balance of ingredients. Serve immediately atop half an orange with segments cut individually, similar to the way one segments a grapefruit. Consume with a shot of cod liver fish oil for optimal health benefits.

Optional: Orange may also be heated.

Caviar Dessert

♦ 4 oz. caviar

♦ ¼ cup whipped raw cream

♦ 1 apple, roughly chopped

✓ Combine caviar and cream.

✓ Use the apple as a cone for your cream scoop. This might seem like a strange ice cream scoop, but in reality, it is very similar. It satisfies you in exactly the same way.

Oriental Dessert

This low-glycemic, creamy fruit can satisfy your dessert cravings.

♦ Quail egg

♦ ⅓ cup cooked white basmati rice

♦ 1 avocado, halved with pit removed

♦ Sea salt and/or torn seaweed sheets

✓ Place quail egg and rice on top of the avocado and serve at room temperature.

Fresh Fruit Sundae

- ◆ 1 banana, peeled and chopped
- ◆ 2 Tbsp sesame, walnut, almond, or coconut oil
- ◆ ⅓ cup fresh berries
- ◆ 1 kiwi, chopped
- ◆ ¼ cup soaked pecans (or nut of your choice)
- ◆ Dash of salt

✓ Combine above ingredients in a bowl. Serve immediately.

Breakfast Entrées Plus

Sweet Potato Breakfast/Dessert

Wild yams are a good way to begin your day.

- 1 wild yam/sweet potato
- 1-2 Tbsp butter oil
- 1 tsp sea salt

✓ Wash yam and add to pot with enough water to half-cover the yams. Steam for 15 min to 1 hour or until soft (depending upon the size of the yam). Serve with oil and salt.

Optional: Add 2 Tbsp berry sauce recipe, which includes a handful of nuts and/or a dash of sea salt. Sprinkle with cloves, cinnamon, nutmeg, and salt. Can serve with spiced season fruit, mylk and coffea drink.

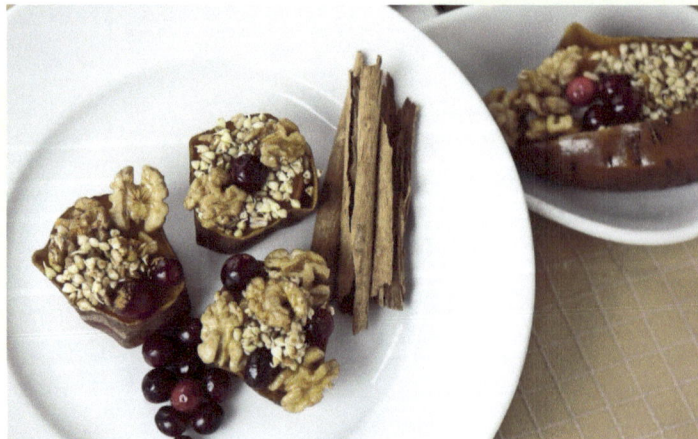

Wild Yam Pie

One and a half days before, soak ⅓ cup wild Irish moss. Eight hours prior, soak ½ cup nuts.

Date paste

- ⅓ cup date paste
- 1 or 2 fresh lemons

Pie Filling

- Meat of 3 young coconuts
- ½ cup water
- ½ cup soaked macadamia nuts
- ⅓ cup soaked wild Irish moss
- 3 steamed & skinned yams
- ½ tsp cloves
- 1 Tbsp cinnamon
- 1 tsp ginger or minced thyme, grated
- 1 tsp sea salt

Date paste: In a food processor, puree 1 Tbsp fresh lemon juice per 5 pitted dates. Set aside.

Pie filling: Blend wild Irish moss, water, soaked nuts, and young coconut meat 11 seconds at a time, allowing mixture to cool in between activity until smooth. Add balance of pie filling ingredients, including date paste, and blend. Pour filling into your favorite crust; allow to set in refrigerator overnight. Serve cold.

Optional: Top pie with candied raisins or candied nuts and mint sprigs.

Egg Punch

- ◆ 1 egg* white
- ◆ 1 Tbsp raw honey
- ◆ 1 egg yolk
- ◆ Orange zest and grated nutmeg
- ◆ 1 peeled and segmented orange or tangerine

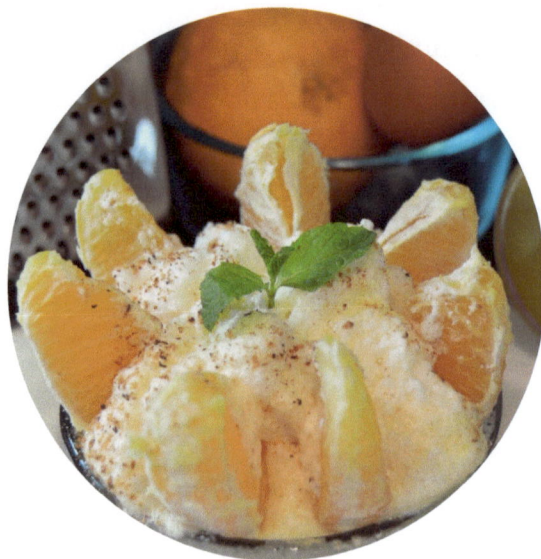

- ✓ Beat egg white until stiff (about 3 minutes). Add raw honey, orange zest, and nutmeg, and beat for 30 seconds. Swirl in egg yolk. Serve with orange or tangerine segments.

*Verify that egg is healthy by confirming that the egg smells good, the egg white looks clear, and the egg yolk sac is strong (doesn't break upon opening). I allow my eggs to get to room temperature before using so that I can better gauge their freshness.

Brie Torte

Eight hours prior, soak ½ cup walnuts.

This makes a great breakfast, dessert, or hors d'oeuvre.

- ◆ ½ cup walnuts, soaked
- ◆ 2 dashes of sea salt, split
- ◆ ⅓ cup local honey

- ◆ 4 oz. traditional goat cheese
- ◆ 1 goat brie or 1 cup goat ricotta
- ◆ ½ cup cranberries, blanched, or pomegranate seeds

✓ Soak nuts. Candy walnut by coating nut with honey and dash of sea salt.

✓ Combine honey, spreadable goat cheese, and a dash of sea salt. Spread creamy goat cheese and honey over round goat brie cheese. Top with nuts and berries. Serve with sliced apples in lemon rub or crackers.

Optional: Replace blanched cranberries with fresh berries, prunes, raisins, or sprouted candied buckwheat groats.

Rice Porridge

♦ 1 cup white basmati rice

♦ 1 can organic coconut milk

✓ Rinse and boil rice in the milk in a covered pot until rice is soft. Serve hot.

Optional: Add soaked raisins and raw local honey and sprinkle with cloves, cinnamon, and nutmeg. Cloves are high in manganese, a much needed nutrient that kills parasites.

Yucca Porridge

Yucca is a natural anti-inflammatory. A good yucca is white upon opening as opposed to speckled.

✓ Substitute peeled yucca for rice in recipe above.

White Bean Blondie and Maca Mylk (recipe follows)

Eight hours prior, soak 1 cup white beans or Great Northern beans. Discard water and boil beans until tender.

- 1 cup boiled beans
- 2 eggs
- ¼ cup coconut butter (you can get this in the shape of a bar of soap cheaply at an Indian, Jamaican, or other ethnic grocer)
- 1 ripe plantain, peeled

- ¾ cup plantain flour
- 1 tsp non-aluminum baking soda
- 1 tsp sea salt
- ½ tsp vanilla flavor
- ½ cup raw sugar
- Jelly of choice

✓ Using a hand mixer, combine above ingredients except jelly. Pour into greased bread loaf mold, swirl in jelly, and bake at 300°F for 30-plus minutes until knife exits clean. Serve hot with a cold glass of maca mylk.

Maca Mylk

- ¼ cup hemp seed
- 1½ cup water
- 1 Tbsp raw coconut nectar/local honey

- ½ tsp maca
- 1 Tbsp mesquite powder
- ½ tsp sea salt

✓ Blend above ingredients into a frothy mixture. Serve at room temperature or cold with crushed ice.

Gluten-Free Plantain/Banana Bread

Optional: Eight hours prior, soak ½ cup pecans or walnuts.

Leave two eggs and a half stick of butter out of the fridge

Flour

- 1 cup plantain flour
- 1½ cup prunes without preservatives (I like the canned Sun Sweet brand.)

- ✓ Combine the above ingredients and use a coffee grinder to create sweetened flour. Yields 2½ cups of sweetened flour.

Dry Ingredients

- Sweetened flour
- ½ tsp salt
- ¼ tsp aluminum free baking soda
- ¼ tsp baking powder

- ✓ Preheat conventional oven to 325°F, and then combine and sift dry ingredients into a bowl.

Wet Ingredients

- 4 Tbsp butter
- ½ cup walnut oil
- 2 eggs
- 4-6 plantains (or 7-9 bananas)

- ✓ In a separate bowl, use a hand blender to combine wet ingredients. Add dry ingredients to wet ingredients a third at a time and mix. Fold in nuts (optional). Bake until bread is fragrant and knife comes out clean, about 40 minutes.

Warm Salad

In order to convert any salad into a meal, just top with anything hot. I mean ANYTHING. It can be split pea soup, lentils, black-eyed pea soup, pinto bean soup, chili, hot fish, hot chicken, hot sausage, hot cauliflower, artichoke, yellow squash casserole, any other casserole, marinara sauce, or large chunks of carrot (so that the carrot is hot while still crunchy). Create a salad with a full complement of beans, sprouts, greens, and fruit.

In order to make your salad nutritionally complete and to make a meal, you want to add some diverse flavors. Foods like basil, parsley, cilantro, scallions, red pepper flakes, fruits, beans, and vegetables improve your culinary experience. Every whole food has a bitter and pungent part, which usually gets cut off and discarded. Do yourself a favor and use every part of the food you use, including the seeds of the tomato, the stems of the parsley, the white vein inside your pepper, the belly button of your carrot, and so forth.

An old recipe for iron deficiency (anemia) is to delete dairy from your diet and drink raw liver drink first thing in the morning when necessary, usually about once per month. Raw liver drink recipe: Blend raw, organic chicken liver, handful of blackberries, and ¼ cup filtered water. Drink immediately.

Soups

Chicken Gizzard Soup

Chicken gizzards are a good source of choline, a brain nutrient, and minerals.

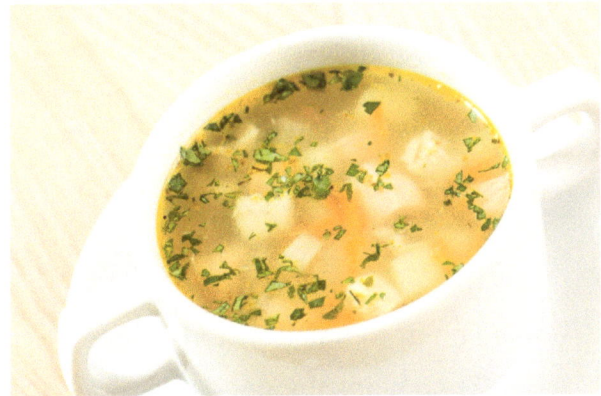

- 1 whole chicken with gizzards
- 4 cups water
- 10 sprigs thyme
- 7 sage leaves
- Salt and pepper to taste

✓ Rinse gizzards and chicken with filtered water. Remove breast and save for another recipe. Remove skin from chicken (toast and give to pet). Place ingredients in pot and boil until chicken meat is soft and falls off bone.

Autumn Butternut Soup

The raw greens in this recipe give the enzymes necessary to help with absorption of all nutrients found in the soup.

- 3 cups broken bone soup or chicken broth
- ¼ cup raw light cream
- Meat of chicken, leg or thigh
- 1 butternut squash, peeled with seeds removed

- 8 sprigs or more marjoram (This is the secret ingredient.)
- ¼ cup onion, minced
- 1 garlic clove
- 1 stalk celery, chopped
- Boston lettuce leaves

✓ Simmer ingredients in covered pot until squash is soft. Allow to cool and blend to desired consistency (either lumpy or smooth works). Serve soup hot in bowl over Boston lettuce leaves.

Optional: Add meat of 2 king crab legs.

Broken Bone Soup

Cook time: 18 hours

- Chicken or turkey bones (raw or already baked)
- 1 gallon filtered water
- Juice from half a lemon or lime
- 1 Tbsp black pepper corns

- 2 carrots
- 4 celery stalks
- 5-7 parsley stems
- 3 thyme branches

✓ Boil chicken bones in 1 gallon of filtered water with juice of 1 lemon or lime for 18 hours. To season broth, remove bones and boil with balance of ingredients.

Soups are very healthy and satisfying. These broths make a great base for any of the following soups: minestrone, escarole soup, chicken soup, potato leek soup, pumpkin soup, butternut squash soup, Thai tom yum soup, and so forth. It's important to note that animals often store toxins, such as lead, in their bones. If you can't be sure the animals were healthy, then avoid cooking the bones.

Hot Mineral Broth

This recipe is great way to obtain the vitamins and minerals available in sea vegetables.

- ◆ 1 quart filtered water
- ◆ 1" square of kelp leaf

- ✓ Simmer kelp leaf on low for 20-30 minutes.

Optional: Chipotle adds spicy flavor that masks the seaweed flavor very effectively.

Collagen Broth

- ◆ 1 quart filtered water
- ◆ 5-7 chicken feet
- ◆ Salt & pepper to taste

- ✓ Simmer for 45 minutes. Season with salt & pepper.

Vegan Sancocho (two parts)

I'm Latin, and as a child, I'd eat a hot bowl of oxtail soup with yucca and plantain floating inside.

Broth

- ♦ 3 cups broken bone soup, hot mineral broth, or collagen broth
- ♦ 3 small potatoes, red and white
- ♦ 1 yucca, peeled and cubed
- ♦ 1 green plantain, peeled and cubed
- ♦ ¼ tsp turmeric
- ♦ Pinch of cayenne pepper

✓ Simmer all ingredients in broth and cook until vegetables are soft. Serve with a spoonful of Cilantro Ceviche (recipe below).

Cilantro Ceviche

- ♦ 1 tomato, cubed
- ♦ ¼ cup red onion, chopped
- ♦ ¼ cup cilantro, chopped
- ♦ 1 avocado, cubed
- ♦ ¼ cup water
- ♦ 1 Tbsp lemon juice
- ♦ 1 tsp sea salt

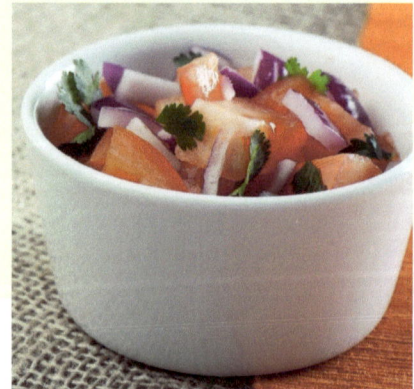

✓ Prepare vegetables and combine all ingredients in a bowl.

Red Lentil Soup

This recipe gives us high amounts of phosphorous that our bodies require. Phosphorous is the second most abundant mineral found in the body.

- ♦ 1 cup red lentils
- ♦ 1½ cups water
- ♦ 1 Tbsp unrefined mustard seed oil
- ♦ 1 large carrot, chopped small
- ♦ ¼ cup fennel, chopped small
- ♦ ¼ cup celery, chopped small
- ♦ Salt & pepper to taste

✓ Rinse and boil lentils with carrot, fennel, and celery in water until tender. Remove from heat and add mustard seed oil and salt. Serve hot with a side of salad.

Black-Eyed Pea Soup with Kaffir Lime Rice

This rice and black-eyed peas dish is so fragrant and delicious. Wow! The secret ingredient is the kaffir leaves.

- ♦ 1 cup black-eyed peas
- ♦ 2½ cups water
- ♦ 1 chipotle
- ♦ 1 inch dried kelp

- ♦ 1 tsp sage leaves, minced
- ♦ 1 tsp thyme
- ♦ 1 tsp rosemary
- ♦ 1 large fennel, cubed

Rice:

- 1 cup white basmati rice, washed
- 1¾ cup water
- 1 tsp oil
- 4 kaffir leaves

✓ In a pot, boil beans in water with chipotle and kelp until soft. Remove black-eyed peas from heat and season with minced sage, thyme, and rosemary. Add fennel (large chop).

Rice: Rinse and boil rice in water with oil and kaffir leaves. Rice is ready when water has evaporated and rice is tender.

Raw Celery Root and Apple

This recipe is delicious. The celery root helps evacuate trapped sodium from the body, something that's much needed for Americans today.

Four to six hours prior, soak 1 cup macadamia nuts.

- 1 cup macadamia nuts
- ¼ cup water
- 1 small celery root, peeled and cubed
- 1 large or 2 small apples
- Lemon rind, grated
- Salt & pepper to taste

✓ Blend nuts with water until mixture reaches desired consistency. Add remaining ingredients and blend until mixed. Serve in bowl with a swirl of olive or truffle oil. A tri-color salad makes a nice side.

Dips

Dips are a great way to eat raw vegetables in a satisfying way. Here are some dip ideas you will absolutely enjoy.

Raw Vegetable Dips

Sunflower Pate

One hour prior, soak raw sunflower seeds in water.

- 1 cup sunflower seeds, soaked
- 1 tsp miso
- 1 Tbsp apple cider vinegar, raw
- ¼ cup dill, chopped
- ¼ cup unrefined olive oil
- Salt, pepper, and red pepper flakes to taste

Optional: 2-4 oz. broiled/grilled salmon

- ✓ Add all ingredients to a food processor and blend to desired consistency.
- ✓ Serve with a side of raw vegetables like zucchini, yellow squash, carrots, celery sticks, cherry tomatoes, and romaine hearts

Salmon Dip

- 5 oz. wild salmon, baked
- 7 oz. sheep yogurt
- 1 tsp horseradish
- 1 Tbsp cod liver fish oil
- Salt & pepper to taste

✓ Add all ingredients to a food processor and blend to desired consistency.
✓ Serve with a platter of chopped raw vegetables.

Sweet Dip

- 1 organic ripe avocado, pitted and peeled
- 1 ripe pear, mashed
- 1 Tbsp raw coconut butter
- ¼ tsp minced jalapeno pepper
- Salt & pepper to taste

✓ Add all ingredients to a food processor and blend to desired consistency. This is good as a vegetable dip or with potato or corn chips.

Raw Vegetable Dip

Sheep's yogurt gives our body essential amounts of B-12, rarely found in the vegan world.

- ◆ 1 cup sheep yogurt
- ◆ 1 avocado
- ◆ 1 Tbsp sage
- ◆ 1 Tbsp thyme

- ◆ 1 Tbsp basil
- ◆ ¼ tsp oregano
- ◆ ¼ tsp jalapeno pepper
- ◆ Salt & pepper

✓ Add all ingredients to a food processor and blend to desired consistency. Serve with a raw vegetable platter.

Cream of Dill Dip

- ◆ ½ cup dill
- ◆ ¼ cup parsley
- ◆ Coin of horseradish
- ◆ 1 Tbsp sour cream
- ◆ 1 Tbsp homemade mayo (see recipe page 120)

- ◆ 1 Tbsp raw apple cider vinegar
- ◆ ½ Tbsp honey
- ◆ ¼ shallot
- ◆ ¼ tsp mustard seed
- ◆ Salt & pepper to taste

✓ Add all ingredients to a food processor and blend to desired consistency. Serve with a raw vegetable platter.

Pinto Bean Dip (2 parts)

Soak 1 cup pinto beans overnight. Discard water in the morning.

- ♦ 1 lb. pinto beans
- ♦ ¼ tsp turmeric
- ♦ ¼ tsp cumin

✓ Place beans in a covered pot with enough water to cover beans fully. Add turmeric and cumin and boil until soft, about 30 minutes. Add to Raw Salsa below.

Raw Salsa

- ♦ 1 scallion, minced
- ♦ 1 garlic tooth, creamed*
- ♦ 1 tomato, finely chopped
- ♦ Beans at room temperature

- ♦ ½ tsp red palm oil**
- ♦ 2 Tbsp olive oil
- ♦ Salt & pepper to taste

✓ In a separate pan, simmer tomatoes in 1 Tbsp of olive oil until soft. Using a food processor or blender, puree soft beans and cooked tomato along with above ingredients until creamy. Serve alongside raw vegetable platter.

* To cream a tooth of garlic, mash with the side of your knife, and cover with olive oil and sea salt. Allow to sit for 3 minutes.

** Red palm oil has a distinct flavor that can be difficult for Westerners. I recommend looking for a brand like Nutiva that has worked to reduce the strong scent while keeping as many of the nutrients as possible.

Salad Dressing Recipes

Enrichment Regarding Unrefined Oils

Be sure to purchase your oils with a freshness date on them so you know they are not processed. So many books have been published on the coconut oil, butter oil, red palm oil, olive oil, and Siberian pine nut oil "miracles." All fresh oils heal the body. Unrefined oils are terrific building blocks that we can build a healthy brain, nervous system, and hormones from, as well as clean our liver and arteries. A word of caution about unrefined soy, canola, corn, and safflower oils, though. Hundreds of studies confirm these oils tend to be very unstable and become rancid even prior to being bottled.

Salad dressing and mayonnaise present opportunities to consume unrefined oils and other fresh ingredients. YouTube has great videos on how to make your own mayonnaise using unrefined olive oil as opposed to low-grade vegetable oil. A great idea is to add 2 to 3 ounces of unrefined Siberian pine nut oil to your 33-ounce bottle of unrefined olive oil. Siberian pine nut oil contains a potent antioxidant and stimulates abundant duodenal release of cholecystokinin (CCK), a catalyst for proper digestion of food in the intestinal tract, allowing you to extract more nutrients from your meal.

Dressing recipes

Coconut

- ¼ cup olive oil
- 1 tsp raw coconut nectar
- 1 tsp parsley
- 1 tsp basil
- Squeeze of lemon or lime
- ¼ tsp salt

✓ Combine ingredients in a food processor and pulse until well combined.

Optional: Follow the above directions for each of the sets of ingredients below for different flavors.

Sesame Honey

- ¼ cup sesame oil
- 1 tsp local honey
- 1 tsp Mrs. Bragg's Liquid Aminos
- ½ tsp tamarind concentrate
- 1 creamed garlic tooth
- ¼ tsp mustard
- dash of salt

Walnut Raspberry

- ¼ cup walnut oil
- ¼ cup raspberries
- 1 tsp honey
- ¼ tsp salt

Walnut Cranberry

- ¼ cup walnut oil
- ¼ cup blanched cranberries
- 1 tsp raw honey
- ¼ tsp salt

Honey Orange

- ¼ cup olive oil
- 1 peeled orange
- 1 tsp raw honey
- 1 tsp mustard
- 1 garlic tooth, creamed
- ¼ tsp salt
- Red pepper flakes

Honey Apple

- ¼ cup olive oil
- 1 tsp yacon syrup/raw honey
- 1 capful raw apple cider vinegar
- 1 tsp rosemary
- 1 tsp thyme
- ¼ tsp salt

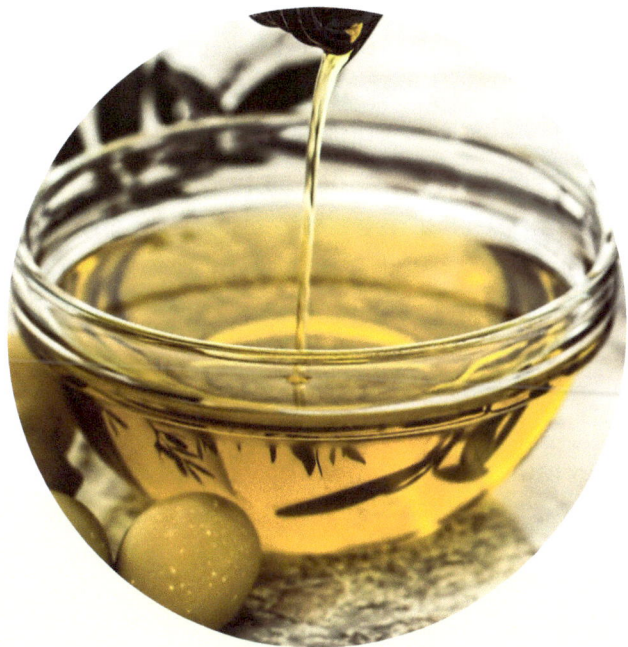

Creamy Dressings

Homemade mayo provides an opportunity to not only eat raw egg but also helps us avoid commercial mayo made from vegetable oils such as soybean and canola. These rancid fats create hormonal imbalance by adding estrogenic foods to our diet, as mentioned in *Anti-Estrogenic Diet* by Ori Hofmekler.

My travels have shown me that, in many countries, eggs are not placed in the refrigerator. Today, I make a practice of leaving the number of eggs my family consumes in a given week out on the counter so that they will act their age when I go to use them. The cold can mask undesirable qualities.

In Asia, breakfast consists of rice, shredded seaweed sheets, and a raw chicken or quail egg. As long as we take the proper precautions, eating raw, healthy eggs is excellent for your health, as many nutrients, such as choline, are lost in the cooking process. Thousands around the globe consume raw eggs.

Homemade Mayonnaise

All ingredients should be at room temperature before starting recipe.

- ¾ cup olive oil
- Twist of lemon
- 1 tsp sea salt
- 1 whole egg
- 1 egg yolk
- ¼ tsp mustard

✓ Add twist of lemon and salt to oil and set aside. Add egg, yolk, and mustard to bowl. Whisk (or use hand blender) until blended and bright yellow. Add oil very slowly, whisking constantly. Use a few drops at a time for the first 4 minutes. Add remaining oil in a very slow stream, about 8 minutes. Mayonnaise will be thick and lighter in color.

I recommend you use free videos online to learn exactly how to make mayonnaise. Some people can make it in a food processor. I had better luck using a hand blender.

Rosemary Garlic Mayonnaise

Rosemary creates an alpha wave pattern in the wave as opposed to an erratic wave pattern.

- 1 cup homemade mayonnaise recipe
- 1 tsp minced rosemary
- 1 garlic tooth, creamed

✓ Puree all ingredients in a food processor.

Anchovies Mayonnaise

Anchovies are a great source of B-12, commonly missing from our everyday diet.

- 1 cup homemade mayonnaise recipe
- 1 can anchovies
- ¼ cup Pecorino Romano

✓ Puree all ingredients in a food processor.

Honey Horseradish Mayonnaise

Horseradish evacuates the free radicals created in our bodies when we eat animal products. This dressing is great with steak. Make your own favorite Thousand Island, Italian herb, ranch, blue cheese, hummus, avocado, and carrot/miso dressing this same way.

- 1 cup homemade mayonnaise recipe
- 1 Tbsp horseradish, grated
- ⅛ tsp raw honey

✓ Puree all ingredients in a food processor.

Salads Plus

These foods are considered fat burn foods because they stimulate metabolism. This salad should be a staple in everyone's diet, as it aids in digestion and helps to eliminate free radicals. For this reason, it is especially complimentary to meals with a lot of red meat and sausage.

Fat Burn Salad

Quantities will vary based on which vegetables you use and how many you need to serve.

Select some or all of the vegetables below:

- Red cabbage
- Green cabbage
- Carrots
- Radishes
- Turnips
- Asparagus
- Celery
- Beets
- Mushrooms
- Brussels sprouts
- Tomatoes
- Juice of ½ lemon or lime
- ½ tsp sea salt

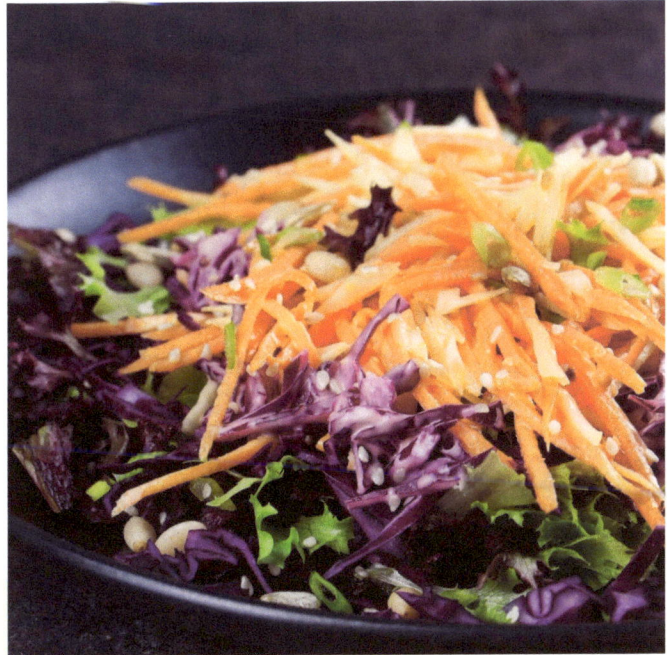

✓ Finely chop any combination of the above vegetables and mix. Add water to midpoint of salad mound. Add lemon or lime juice and salt. Mix again to coat all vegetables. Serve at room temperature.

Optional: Convert recipe to fat burn soup by cooking above ingredients in water (3 cups per person). Serve warm.

Bok Choy Salad

This recipe tastes particularly good with my Shrimp with Shell recipe or sea scallops.

- 2 cup bok choy greens, chopped
- 1 cup cilantro, chopped
- ¼ cup scallion, chopped

Salad Dressing:
- ¼ cup unrefined sesame oil
- 1 tsp rice white vinegar
- 1 tsp Mrs. Bragg's Liquid Aminos
- 1 tsp local honey
- Salt & pepper to taste
- Grated ginger

Optional: jalapeño pepper to taste and/or green papaya. Napa cabbage can be substituted for bok choy.

- ✓ Wash bok choy and cut in half from top to bottom. Then, cut green leaves on the bias. Chop cilantro and scallion. Combine with bok choy. Mix all dressing ingredients and toss with the salad. Serve at room temperature.

Hot Cauliflower (winter option)

This is the far side of salad dressing. Eating hot/cooked and cold/raw is the most satisfying and healthy experience one can have with food. Put this hot cauliflower casserole on your salad instead of dressing. Its creamy consistency makes it a perfect salad dressing in the winter.

- 1 cauliflower
- ½ cup Pecorino Romano cheese
- ¼ cup raw unflavored sheep yogurt
- 1 tsp red palm oil
- 1 tsp red pepper flakes
- Salt & pepper to taste

✓ Quarter cauliflower and lightly steam. Mix together remaining ingredients and place cheese mixture over cauliflower. Bake for 30 minutes at 300F°. Serve hot cauliflower casserole over mixed greens or as a side with dinner.

Red Beet Ravioli (two parts)

Beets are a blood cleanser. Note: Beets can make your stool red.

Nut Cream

Eight hours prior, soak 1 cup macadamia or almond nuts.

- 1 cup soaked nuts
- 2 Tbsp water
- Dash of salt

Raviolis (Beets)

- 1 cup red beets, thinly sliced
- 1 tsp olive oil
- 1 tsp fresh lemon juice
- Dash of salt

Nut cream: Using a high-powered blender, blend above ingredients until creamy, about 11 seconds. Set aside to stuff raviolis.

Raviolis: Marinate beets in oil, lemon juice, and salt. Allow to sit for 15 minutes. Make raviolis with two slices of beet and 1 tsp nut cream between the slices. Sprinkle with minced parsley stems and serve at room temperature.

Optional: White Ravioli

Substitute thinly sliced chayote for beets. For contrast, color the nut cream with fresh, pressed beet or carrot juice for the white ravioli recipe.

Raw Potato Salad

- 2 cup jicama, cubed
- ¼ cup homemade mayo
- 1 Tbsp red onion
- 1 Tbsp parsley, chopped

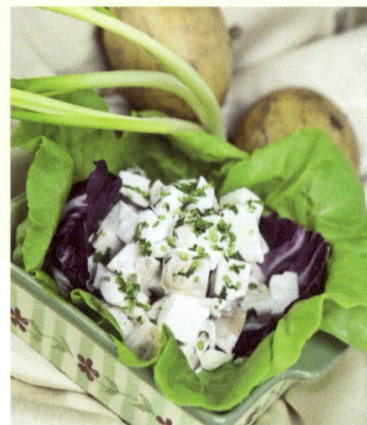

- ✓ Prepare jicama and mix cubes with remaining ingredients. Serve atop marinated greens. This recipe goes well with the Raw Pea Salad recipe below.

Raw Pea Salad

One day prior, sprout fresh peas or purchase pea shoots.

Topping:

- 2 medium carrots, steamed
- 1 tsp brown sugar
- Pea sprouts

Greens Marinade:

- ¼ cup unrefined olive oil
- 1 tsp red wine vinegar
- 1 tsp honey or sweetener
- Salt & pepper to taste

Greens:

- 1 cup spinach
- 2 cups arugula
- 2 cups baby greens

✓ Steam carrots by placing carrots, ½ cup water, and brown sugar in covered pot and simmer until soft, about 15 minutes. In a bowl, mix together ingredients of greens marinade. Toss greens in greens marinade and top with carrots and pea shoots.

Serve on platter at room temp. Your guests will love the flavor and colors.

Raw Tabouli Salad

Celery, an ingredient in this recipe, is a miracle food because it increases blood flow to the brain and body by opening up tiny capillaries that might have become obstructed. Fresh, pressed celery is a wonderful, low-glycemic base for any smoothie, a natural form of salt, and a great aphrodisiac. Mineral salts are important to keep high, especially when transitioning to a natural diet from one that is high in processed foods, which is very high in sodium and low in the 77 other minerals the body requires.

- 1 cup hempseeds, shelled
- 2 Tbsp scallion, finely chopped
- ¼ cup celery, chopped
- ¼ cup parsley
- ¼ cup cilantro (or basil)
- 1 tsp lemon juice
- 1 tsp olive oil
- ⅛ tsp lemon rind, grated
- Pinch of cayenne pepper
- Salt & pepper to taste

✓ Combine all ingredients and serve over a bed of Boston or romaine lettuce.

Fragrant Quinoa

- 1 cup cooked quinoa
- ¼ cup pear, chopped (pear or apple in the winter and mango in the summer)
- ¼ cup parsley
- 1 carrot, chopped
- 1 celery, chopped

Dressing:

- ¼ cup olive oil
- ¼ cup freshly squeezed orange juice
- ¼ tsp freshly squeezed lemon juice
- 1 tsp raw honey
- ⅛ tsp ground allspice
- ⅛ tsp lemon peel, grated
- Salt & pepper to taste

✓ Boil quinoa in water to cover for 20 minutes or until soft. Mix dressing ingredients together. Toss quinoa with other ingredients and add dressing. Serve at room temperature.

Tuna Salad

Look for low-mercury tuna or bone-in sardines packed in natural oils. Don't drain them. This snack is high in omega-3 fatty acids.

- ½ lb. gluten-free pasta or chayote, spiralized
- 1 tsp unrefined olive oil
- 1 can low-mercury tuna or sardines with bone
- 2 Tbsp fennel/celery, finely chopped
- 2 Tbsp parsley
- 2 Tbsp homemade mayo
- 1 tsp cod liver oil
- Salt and red pepper flakes to taste

✓ Boil gluten-free pasta until soft, and then drain. Rinse with cold water and place back in pot. If you choose to use chayote instead of pasta, put the chayote through a spiralizer. Mix the gluten-free pasta or spiralized chayote with 1 tsp unrefined olive oil and a dash of salt. In a separate bowl, combine rest of ingredients. Serve tuna or sardines over pasta or spiralized chayote.

Pumpkin Seed Spicy Ceviche Salad

- ♦ 1 cup cilantro
- ♦ ½ cup pumpkin seeds, soaked
- ♦ 2 Tbsp lemon
- ♦ ½ Tbsp jalapeno, chopped
- ♦ 1 tsp water
- ♦ Cherry tomatoes

✓ In a food processor, puree all ingredients except tomatoes. Spoon mixture into small tomatoes with seeds removed.

Serve as hors d'oeuvre or side dish.

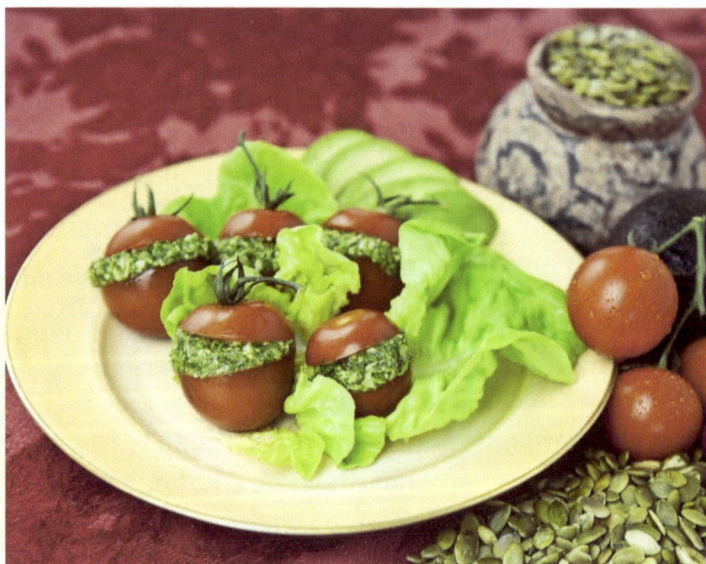

Raw Green Sides

Raw greens are a good way to add raw to your diet, and cooking green vegetables destroys the chlorophyll found in those foods. Chlorophyll oxygenates the body, helps wounds to heal, rids the body of toxic bacteria and body odor, and balances the good bacteria. Try these delicious raw recipes. Greens in general are a great source of vitamin K, protein, and minerals.

Sliced Almonds

Soak sliced almonds for 8 hours.

Broccoli Side

- 3 cup broccoli florets, chopped
- ¼ cup unrefined olive oil
- 1 tsp sea salt
- Almonds, sliced and soaked (amount optional)

✓ Combine ingredients in bowl and mix well. Allow greens to wilt for 30 minutes or so before consuming.

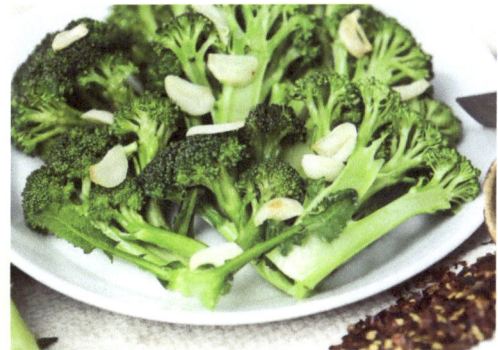

Broccoli is rich in sulforaphane, a nutrient that helps rebuild DNA that has become damaged.

Optional:

- 1 garlic tooth, creamed *
- ¼ cup Pecorino Romano

✓ Add to Broccoli Side and serve.

*To cream a garlic tooth, crush with rock or side of knife, add a few drops of olive oil, and sprinkle with sea salt.

131

Snow Peas

- ¾ cup cooked white basmati rice
- 1 carrot, chopped into cubes
- 2 cups snow peas, washed
- ¼ cup unrefined olive oil
- 1 garlic tooth, creamed
- 1 tsp ginger, grated
- 1 tsp Mrs. Bragg's Liquid Aminos
- ½ cup sesame seeds, soaked for 1 hour
- Salt & black pepper to taste

✓ Rinse rice and put into pot with 1½ cups filtered water. Boil until water has been fully absorbed. Prepare vegetables. Place all ingredients into bowl, and mix fully. Allow to wilt until rice has cooled somewhat. Then add vegetables to the rice. Serve at room temperature.

Asparagus

One day prior, soak raw walnut halves in water for 8 hours and allow to dry.

- 2 cups asparagus, washed and cut in half
- ¼ cup walnuts, sprouted
- ¼ cup unrefined walnut oil
- 1 tsp raw apple cider vinegar
- ½ tsp mustard seed or mustard oil
- Salt and pepper to taste
- Shallots, sliced, quantity to taste

✓ Prepare asparagus. Combine oil, vinegar, mustard, salt, and pepper to make a dressing. Pour over asparagus; allow to wilt about 15 minutes. Toss with shallots. Serve at room temperature.

Kale Salad

- ◆ 3 cups kale
- ◆ 1 yellow squash
- ◆ ¼ cup Pecorino Romano
- ◆ 2 Tbsp water
- ◆ Salt and pepper to taste
- ◆ Dash of cayenne pepper

✓ Wash and tear kale leaves; mince or remove large stems. Add rest of ingredients to food processor and pulse until reach desired consistency. Combine kale and mixture fully. Serve at room temperature.

Summer Collard Salad

- ◆ 5 organic collard green leaves
- ◆ 1 carrot, washed and cut into matchsticks
- ◆ 1 mango, peeled and cubed
- ◆ 1 celery stalk, chopped small
- ◆ ¼ cup unrefined olive oil
- ◆ Salt and pepper to taste

✓ Rinse collard greens, remove vein from collard green, tear leaves, and mince stems. Combine all ingredients in a bowl and allow to wilt for 15 minutes. Serve at room temperature.

Optional: Add sunflower seeds that were soaked for one hour and allowed to dry. Add to rest of salad.

133

Other Sides and Entrées

Pesto Pasta Entrée

Pesto

Soak pumpkin seeds for 1 hour.

- 1 cup basil
- 1 cup parsley
- ¼ cup pumpkin seeds, soaked

- 1 tsp lemon/lime juice
- 1 tsp olive oil
- Dash of salt

✓ Combine ingredients in a food processor and pulse until desired consistency. Sweet potato fries are a great compliment.

Optional: Serve with chopped tomato marinated in 1 tsp olive oil, mashed garlic tooth, and sea salt.

Or serve pesto on top of spiralized zucchini marinated in 1 tsp olive oil, mashed garlic tooth, and dash of sea salt.*

Or serve tomatoes and pesto over gluten-free pasta instead of spiralized zucchini.

Or sprinkle red pepper flakes on the pesto and serve at room temperature.

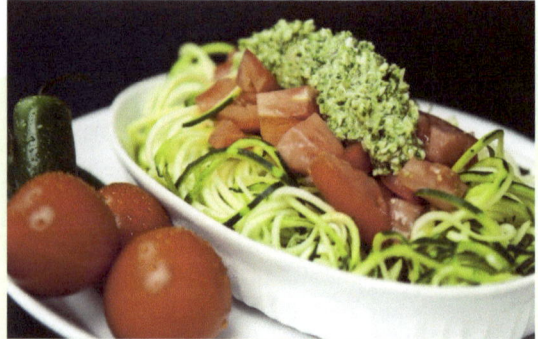

*Eating un-marinated raw vegetables might make you bloated, so marinate!

Raw Mac-n-Cheese

This recipe makes a wonderful side dish any time of year and is a great way to increase the amount of zinc, sulfur, healthy fats, and fiber in your diet if you choose to make your own nut cheese, as sprouted nuts are particularly high in fats that the brain requires for good health. For convenience, use a goat ricotta or Pecorino Romano, which is high in B-12, an essential brain nutrient.

- 2 yellow squash, spiralized
- 1 tsp olive oil
- 2 scallions, chopped
- ¼ cup goat ricotta or nut cheese
- 1 tsp Pecorino Romano
- 1 tsp red pepper flakes
- 1 tsp paprika
- 1 tsp sea salt & pepper

✓ In a bowl, mix olive oil, scallions, cheese, salt, and pepper. Fold in spiralized yellow squash.

An alternative to using a spiralizer is a mandolin or a manual grater.

Optional: Nut Cheese – This step not required if you opt to use cheese.

One day prior, soak macadamia nuts or Marcona almonds for 8 hours, drain, and allow to dry in sieve or open plate for 4 hours.

- ◆ 1 cup macadamia nuts, soaked
- ◆ 1 tsp filtered water
- ◆ 1 tsp sea salt

- ✓ Blend macadamia nuts, 1 Tbsp filtered water, and dash of salt until creamy, about 11 seconds.
- ✓ Serve with a side of steamed cauliflower. To steam cauliflower, simmer cauliflower in covered pot with 1 cup of water and dash of salt until soft, about 30 minutes.

Fries

Fries are a staple in our American diet, and raising the bar on everyday foods is the objective of this book. In an effort to raise the bar on fries, let us expand our notion of fries and upgrade the oil they are fried in. Coating our fries in ¼ cup olive oil and a 1 Tbsp of red palm oil before baking at 400°F raises their nutritional value very effectively. Red palm oil is high in vitamin A, which is very healing for us; and it has a full-spectrum vitamin E, a powerful antioxidant. Here are some ideas for nutrient dense fries.

Sweet Potato Fries

- 3 wild yams
- ¼ cup cooking olive oil
- 1 tsp red palm oil
- Salt & pepper to taste

- ✓ Cut raw sweet potatoes into wedges, coat in oil and salt, lay out on cookie sheet, and bake at 375°F until crisp, about 30 minutes. Allow to cool and harden. Serve at room temperature with dip recipe below.

Sweet Potato Dip

- ⅓ cup unrefined walnut oil
- 1 tsp cinnamon
- Handful of cranberries
- Dash of salt

- ✓ Puree above ingredients in a food processor and serve.

Yucca Fries & Pink Sauce

1-2 yuccas

1 cup cooking olive oil

1 Tbsp red palm oil

Salt to taste

Pink Sauce

- ♦ ¼ cup organic catsup
- ♦ ¼ cup homemade mayonnaise

✓ Purchase yucca that is white on the inside (no dark veins). Peel and cut yucca; then steam in covered pot until soft, about 15 minutes. Fry yucca in oil until crisp on the outside, about 10 minutes. Salt to taste. Serve with side of pink sauce, which consists of homemade mayo and catsup.

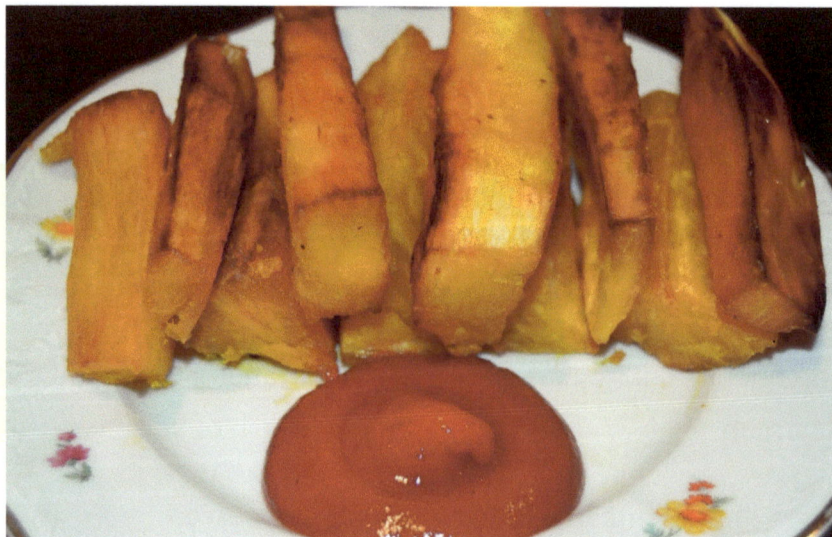

Green Plantain Fries with Guacamole

One hour prior, soak pumpkin seeds.

- 2 large green plantains
- 1 cup olive oil
- 1-2 Tbsp red palm oil
- Sea salt to taste

Guacamole

2-3 ripe avocados, mashed

2 Tbsp pumpkin seeds, soaked

¼ cup cilantro, chopped

1 small tomato, chopped small

1 tsp red onion, minced

1 tsp fresh lime juice

Sea salt & pepper to taste

Peel 2 large green plantains and cut into quarters. Fry in oil until soft in the middle, about 10 minutes. Remove and smash with cooking rock or side of chef's knife. Sprinkle with salt and then fry until crisp, about 10 minutes.

Serve with side of guacamole. Cut avocados in half; remove pit, spoon out flesh, and combine with other ingredients. Serve at room temperature with pit to keep avocado green.

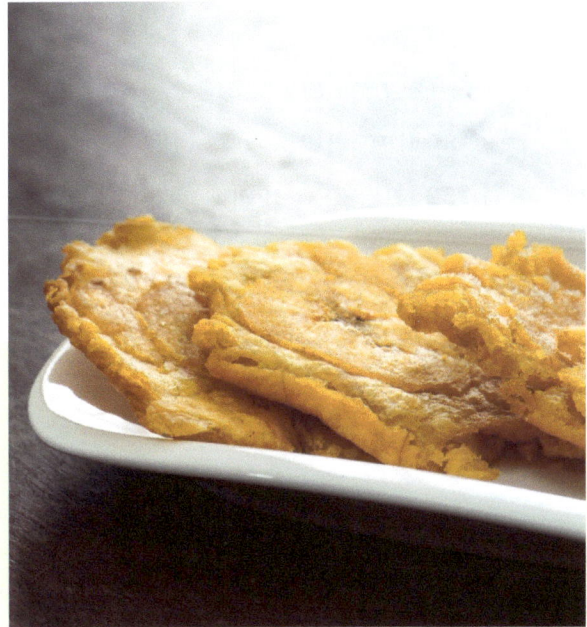

Entrées

Gluten Free Veggie Burger

- 4 large red potatoes
- ⅓ cup Kamut grain
- 3 eggs
- 3 carrots
- 1 large beet
- ¼ cup fennel bulb, minced
- ¼ cup scallions
- 1½ Tbsp celery salt
- 1 tsp turmeric
- 1 tsp jalapeno pepper, minced
- 1 cup olive oil
- 1 tsp red palm oil
- ¼ cup potato, mashed
- 1 Tbsp cooked Kamut
- 1 Tbsp raw carrot, grated
- 1 Tbsp raw beet, grated
- ½ tsp fennel seed, crushed
- 1 tsp celery seed
- Dash of salt
- Dash of turmeric
- 1 tsp scallions, chopped
- ⅛ tsp jalapeño or crushed red pepper flakes

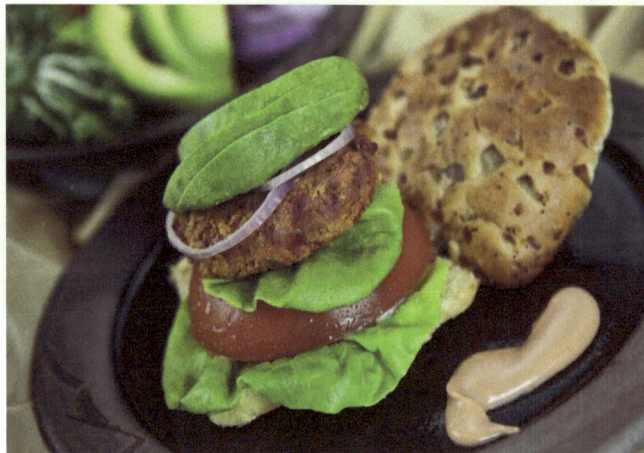

✓ Boil potatoes until soft; then mash and set aside. Rinse and boil Kamut in 1 cup water in covered pot until soft; set aside. Grate carrots and beet, mince fennel, chop scallions, and mince jalapeno pepper. In a separate bowl, beat eggs. Mix all ingredients together. Now you are ready to begin.

✓ Form into thin burgers using your hands. Use egg to help you create patties. Sauté veggie burgers in oil until crisp on the outside; remove from heat with spatula and allow to cool. Set on an open plate. Serve over a bed of romaine or Boston lettuce, sliced avocado, and tomato with a side of pink sauce. These burgers can be frozen and reheated for a quick dinner.

✓ *Or* save yourself work and just use a grilled portobello mushroom coated with olive oil and vinegar or lemon. The easier your diet is, the better, and it's the most delicious burger you'll ever have.

Acorn Entrée

- ◆ 1 acorn squash
- ◆ ½ cup cranberries, blanched
- ◆ ¼ cup butter oil/ghee
- ◆ 1 red apple, cubed
- ◆ Salt to taste

✓ Cut acorn squash in half and scoop seeds out. Place seeds on a separate dish and set aside. Bake acorn halves facedown in baking dish at 350°F until soft. Blanch cranberries by placing cranberries in 2 cups boiling water for 1 minute.

✓ Pour 1½ Tbsp butter oil on each acorn hal, sprinkle with salt, and place apples in crater. Serve faceup.

✓ For an added snack, bake squash seeds at 200°F for 5-10 minutes until crunchy.
Optional: Serve with a side of mushrooms (wild or white button) and Brussels sprouts sautéed in 1 tsp olive oil and 1 tsp red palm oil in a cast iron skillet.

Raw Spaghetti with Vegan Meatballs (5 parts)

Preparing mung bean sprouts takes 1-2 days if you have none on hand. Soak 2 cups raw almonds for 8 hours before cooking.

Meatballs

The meatballs are simply a smaller version of the vegetarian burger above.

Tomato Sauce

- 1- 16 oz. can tomato puree
- 5-10 basil stems
- 1 tsp oregano, minced
- 1 garlic tooth
- 1 small onion
- 1 tsp olive oil

Sprouts

- ½ cup sprouted mung beans

Cheese

- 2 cups soaked almonds
- ¾ cup filtered water

or

- Pecorino Romano cheese

Vegetable Pasta

- 1-2 zucchini
- 1 tsp olive oil
- 1 garlic tooth, creamed
- Salt to taste

Cheese: To prepare almond cheese, soak 2 cups raw almonds for 8 hours. Drain, remove skin, and blend in high-powered blender with ¾ cup water until creamy, about 11 seconds. Repeat 11-second blend cycle if necessary. Add creamed garlic tooth to almond mixture. Or use Pecorino Romano (comes from sheep) as cheese.

Tomato Sauce: In a pan, sauté 1 tsp olive oil and 1 small diced onion until translucent. Then, add tomato puree, tooth of garlic, basil stems, oregano. Cover and simmer for 40 minutes.

Vegetable Pasta: Push a zucchini through a spiralizer to create raw spaghetti. Combine 1 tsp unrefined olive oil and salt to improve the digestibility of zucchini spaghetti.

Sprouts: Adding crunch to pasta dishes is important. I find mung bean sprouts work well. Here are the sprouting instructions again for your convenience. Rinse and soak ½ cup mung beans in 4 cups of filtered water and 1 tsp food-grade hydrogen peroxide in ½ gallon Mason jar covered with cheesecloth for 8-12 hours. Drain, rinse, drain, and lay Mason jar on its side for 8-12 hours. Repeat last step until a tiny root forms, signaling that the bean is enzymatically alive and ready for ingestion.

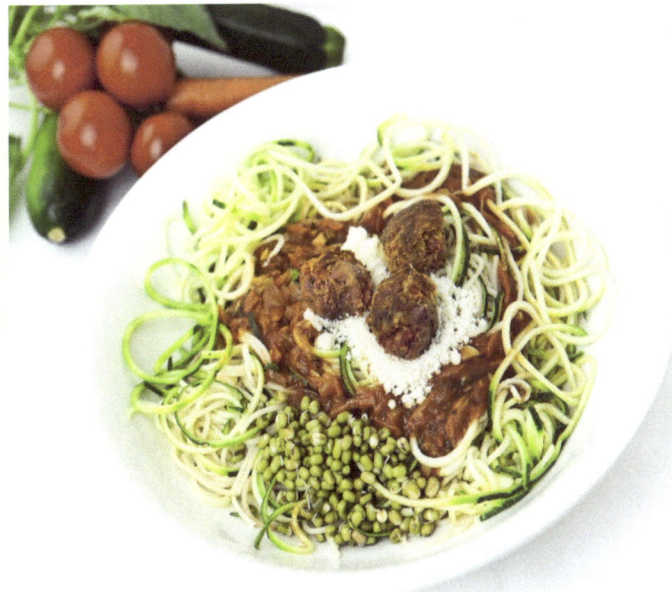

Raw Lasagna

Eight hours before, soak 1 cup raw almonds or macadamia nuts.

Raw Red Sauce

- ½ cup almonds, soaked
- ½ cup filtered water
- ½ cup sun-dried tomatoes
- ¼ cup unrefined olive oil
- 1 Tbsp honey
- 1 tsp sea salt

Green Basil Paste

- 1 cup fresh basil leaves
- ½ cup almonds, soaked
- ½ cup water
- ⅓ cup unrefined olive oil
- ½ tsp amla
- 1 tsp sea salt
- 1 beefsteak tomato

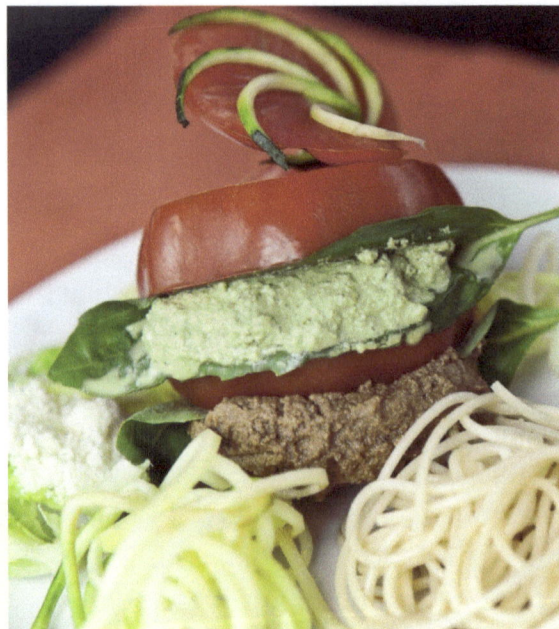

Raw Red Sauce: Soak ½ cup sun-dried tomatoes for 15 minutes (with a few drops of food-grade hydrogen peroxide to kill mold found on all dried fruits); then drain. Using a high-powered blender, combine ½ cup soaked nuts with water and blend until creamy. Add all other red sauce ingredients and puree until creamy, about 11 seconds.

Green Basil Paste: Using a high-powered blender, combine ½ cup soaked nuts with water and blend until creamy. Add all green paste ingredients and puree until creamy, about 11 seconds.

Slice a beefsteak tomato in thirds and place green sauce in one layer and red sauce in another.

Serve at room temperature over a bed of arugula or Boston lettuce.

If you prefer a creamier consistency to the red and green sauce, you may substitute Marcona almonds for regular almonds, but these are more expensive and less readily available.

Collard Greens Parmesan

Marinara Sauce

- 1- 16 oz. can tomato puree
- 1 small yellow onion
- 2 garlic teeth
- 2 Tbsp red palm oil
- 1 tsp oregano
- 5-10 basil stems

Cheese

- 1 steamed cauliflower or 2 yellow squash
- ½ cup Pecorino Romano
- 1 cup goat ricotta
- Salt and pepper to taste

Marinara Sauce: Sauté chopped onions until translucent. Add balance of ingredients, cover pot, and simmer for one hour.

Cheese: Steam cauliflower or 2 yellow squash and mash into balance of cheese mixture ingredients.

Serve warm marinara sauce over raw collard green leaf or bed of basil. Top with cheese mixture and serve warm.

Red meat has many health benefits that many of us never see. Consuming raw meat and fish provides the highest nutrition while prompting you to stop before you have overeaten. Raw fish and meat are very high in tyrosine, the amino acid our bodies make for energy and strength. Many within our society seek for a pick-me-up in caffeine and sugar, when it's tyrosine, found in raw eggs, meat, and fish, where that pick-me-up can best be found.

Raw meat/fish/egg reduces the amount of sex binding globulin in circulation, thus allowing more free testosterone to circulate. This is important because as we age, the amount of free testosterone in our bodies diminishes along with our vitality. Testosterone gives us spatial abilities so that we can judge the space around us, predict our own movement, and participate with certainty in our environment—very helpful for those with ADHD.

Tartare

Steak Tartare

This yields 4 servings. Serve one and freeze other 3 servings for later use. It will taste great any time you thaw it.

- 1 lb. raw, lean, organic beef or ground bison beef, thinly sliced
- ¼ cup unrefined olive oil
- 2 Tbsp red onion, chopped
- 2 Tbsp horseradish, grated
- 1 tsp sea salt
- Pepper to taste

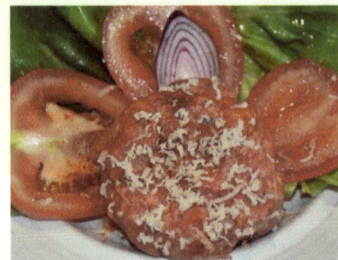

- ✓ Combine above ingredients. Serve over a bed of Boston lettuce, chopped beefsteak tomato, with yucca fries.

Salmon Tartare

This recipe adds much needed omega-3 oils into our diet.

- 1 lb. raw, wild-caught salmon, thinly sliced
- ½ cup dill, chopped
- 2 Tbsp red onion, minced
- 2 Tbsp cod liver fish oil
- 1 tsp sea salt
- 2 Tbsp raw cheese, grated

✓ Combine above ingredients and serve over a bed of arugula and cubed tomato. Serve with a side of yucca fries.

Snapper Tartare

- ¼ lb. snapper fillet, thinly sliced
- 1 tsp cod liver or fish oil
- ¼ cup capers
- 2 Tbsp red onions, sliced
- 1 tsp Mrs. Bragg's Liquid Aminos
- 1 tsp horseradish, grated

✓ Combine above ingredients and serve over a bed of radishes and arugula.

Dirty Rice with Raw Salsa

- ¾ cup white basmati rice
- ½ cup water
- 1 cup organic chicken livers, chopped
- 1 medium onion, chopped
- 1 tsp red palm oil
- 1 tsp olive oil

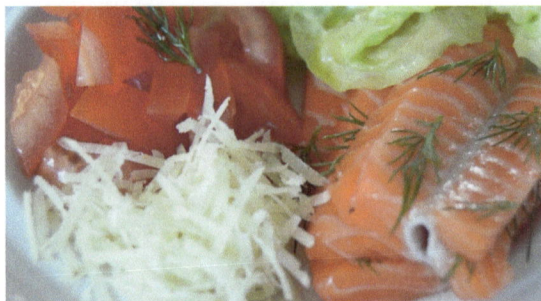

Raw Salsa

- 2 celery stalks, minced
- ½ cup jalapeno pepper with the seeds, chopped
- 1 green pepper, seeded and chopped
- 1 tsp oregano
- ½ tsp drop of Mrs. Bragg's Liquid Aminos
- ½ tsp turmeric
- ½ tsp cumin

✓ Rinse and boil white basmati rice in water and cover. Rice is ready when water has been absorbed and rice is soft.

✓ Sauté chicken livers and onion in red palm oil and olive oil for 15 minutes or until chicken livers are pink in the middle.

✓ Mix raw salsa ingredients. Combine rice, chicken livers, and raw salsa. Serve hot over a bed of Boston lettuce and sliced tomatoes.

Black-Eyed Pea Soup with Rice and Collard Greens

This makes a great side to any BBQ dinner. Baked plantains also go especially well with black-eyed peas.

Bean Soup

- 1 cup dried black-eyed peas
- 1 cup filtered water
- 12 oz. can organic diced tomatoes
- 1 tsp olive oil
- 1 tooth garlic
- ½ cup water
- 1 onion
- 1 tsp green chilies or jalapeno peppers
- 3 bay leaves
- 1 large carrot, chopped
- 1 celery stalk, chopped
- 1 tsp jalapeño pepper

Rice

- ¾ cup rinsed basmati white rice
- 1½ cups filtered water
- *Optional*: kaffir lime leaves

Greens

- Collard green leaves
- Unrefined olive oil
- Sea salt

Bean Soup: Sauté yellow onion, carrot, celery stalk, and jalapeño pepper in 1 tsp olive oil until translucent. Rinse black-eyed peas and add to onions with water and balance of ingredients. Simmer until beans become soft, about 40 minutes.

Rice: Rinse basmati white rice and boil in 1½ cups water in covered pot until water has been absorbed and rice is soft.

Collard Greens: Remove vein and rub salt and oil on leaves.

Serve beans and rice with collard green leaves.

Optional: Top with grated raw spicy jack and/or hot red sauce.

Shrimp with Shell

This recipe is high in glucosamine, important for joint health.

- 1 lb. shrimp with shell
- 1 tsp red palm oil
- ¼ cup olive oil
- 1 garlic tooth
- Salt and pepper to taste

✓ Sauté shrimp in oil and garlic until crisp. Season with salt and pepper.
✓ Serve with a side of greens rubbed in unrefined olive oil and salt, white button mushrooms, corn, chopped tomatoes, and shallots.

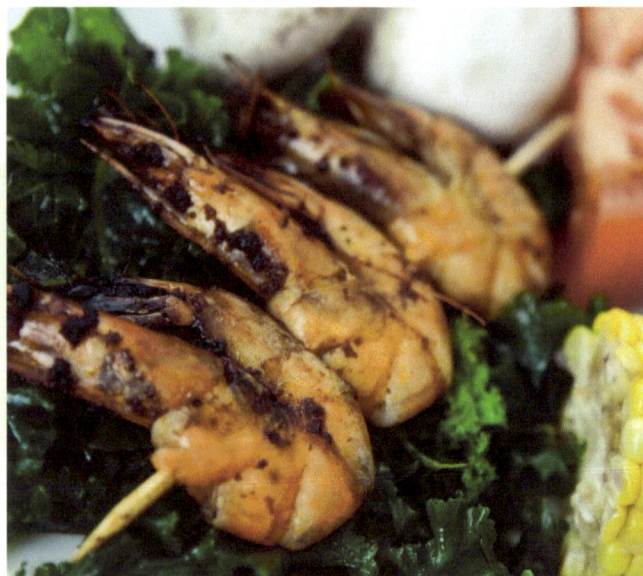

Red Yeast Rice Meatloaf

This meatloaf recipe is high in beta-carotene, fiber, and B vitamins. Meat is nourishing when it is a small part of a meal.

Rice Mixture

- ¾ cup white basmati rice
- 1½ cup of water
- 1 tsp red yeast rice
- 1 tsp red palm oil
- 1 tsp salt

Beef Mixture

- 2 lbs. ground beef or ground bison
- ¼ cup scallion, chopped
- 1- 16 oz. can tomato puree
- 3 eggs
- 1 cup Pecorino Romano
- 1 capful raw apple cider vinegar
- 1 tsp oregano, chopped
- 3 garlic cloves, mashed
- 1 tsp cumin
- 1 tsp turmeric

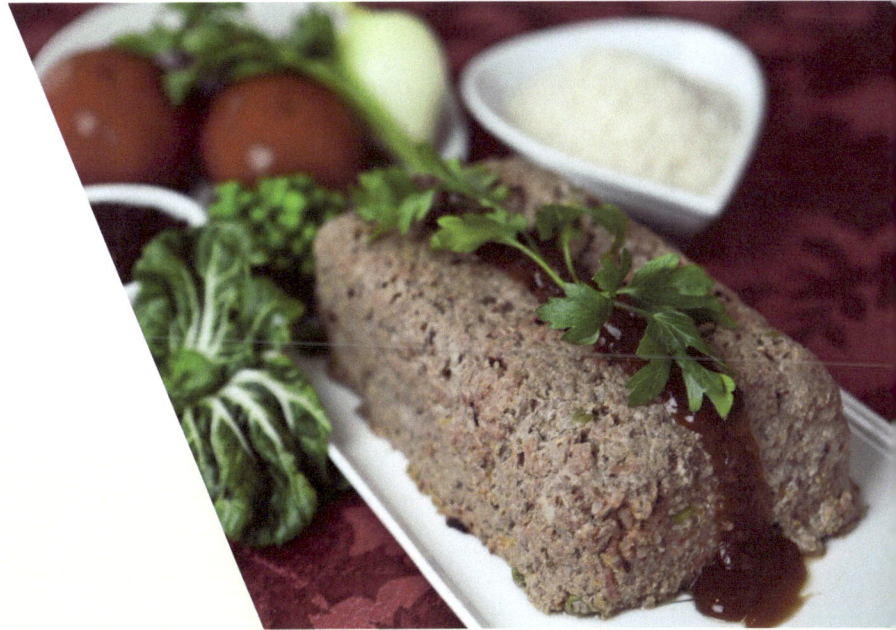

Rice: Bring rice to a rolling boil; then add red yeast rice, cover, and simmer until water has been removed and rice is soft.

Meatloaf: Combine rice and beef mixture in a large bowl. Place mixture into 2 baking dishes (I usually freeze one) and bake at 350°F for 30 minutes until fragrant. Salt is a living food so add salt at the table and remember that Pecorino Romano is salty.

Serve with salad, sautéed vegetables, Pecorino Romano, pasta, and marinara sauce. Remember that your pasta can be a spiralized zucchini or chayote in olive oil and salt rub.

Vegetarian Tacos

One day prior, sprout quinoa per instructions provided.

Eight hours prior, soak pinto beans.

One hour prior, soak sunflower seeds and pumpkin seeds.

Raw Taco Meat
- 1 cup sprouted quinoa
- 1 cup sunflower seeds, soaked
- ½ Tbsp blackstrap molasses
- ¼ cup raw, local honey
- 2 Tbsp unrefined olive oil
- 1 tsp cumin
- ½ tsp turmeric
- 2 Tbsp chopped scallion/leek
- ½ tsp oregano, minced
- Salt and pepper to taste

Beans

- 1 cup pinto beans
- 1 yellow onion
- 1 large tomato
- 1 tsp finely chopped parsley stems
- 1 tsp cumin
- ½ tsp turmeric

Raw Taco Meat: One day prior, sprout quinoa in ½ gallon Mason jar following sprouting instructions at the start of the recipes section. One hour prior, soak sunflower seeds. Combine balance of veggie meat ingredients and use as seasoning for sprouted grains and seeds.

Beans: Eight hours prior, soak pinto beans. After eight hours, drain beans, place in pot, and add water to cover, with a dash of turmeric and cumin. Cover and boil until soft; then remove from heat to cool. In a pan, sauté onions, parsley stems, and tomato until onions become translucent. Add to hot beans during last 5 minutes of cooking or once they have been removed from heat.

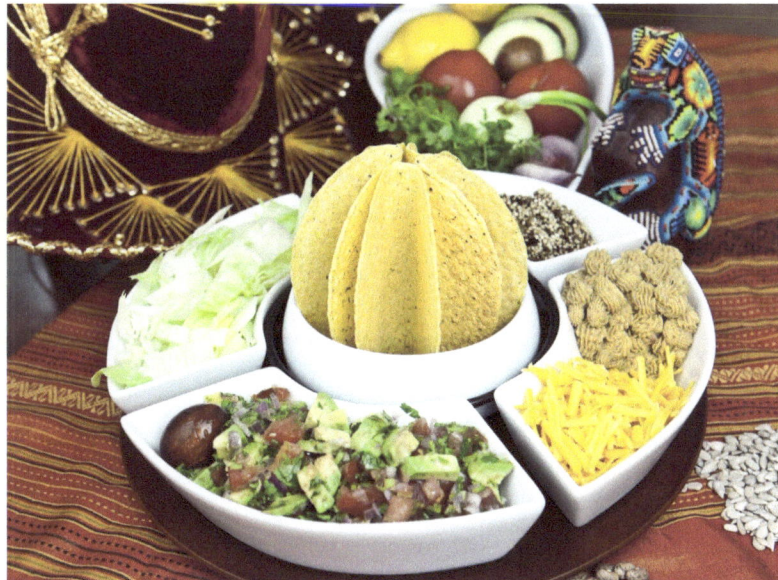

Guacamole Side

- 2-3 ripe avocados
- 2 Tbsp hulled pumpkin seeds (aka pepitas), soaked
- ¼ cup chopped cilantro
- 1 small tomato, minced
- 1 tsp red onion, minced
- 1 tsp fresh lime juice
- Sea salt to taste

✓ For one hour, soak pumpkin seeds. Cut avocados in half; remove pit, spoon out flesh, and combine with other ingredients. Serve at room temperature with pit to keep guacamole green.

✓ Serve with grated cheese, chopped lettuce, and taco shells.

Sushi

Sushi (Three parts)

Horseradish pushes blood to the brain while ginger pushes blood to our extremities, keeping all areas fully oxygenated and vibrant. I love this recipe because it is high in fiber, and sea vegetables are a natural blue food, meaning they are rich in calcium, a source of lean protein, and full of minerals and B vitamins. Plus, it's tantalizing to the palate.

Miso Soup

- 1 square inch of kelp
- 1 tsp miso
- 3 cups water
- 1 white button mushroom, thinly sliced
- ½ scallion, finely chopped

✓ Simmer water and kelp for 20 minutes. Remove kelp leaf or mince and keep in soup. Remove from heat; add miso, mushroom, and scallion. Serve warm.

Sushi

- 1 large carrot, steamed
- 1 ripe avocado

Optional: salmon

✓ Steam carrot. Pit avocado and cube flesh.

Perfect Sushi Rice

- 2 parsnips
- 1 tsp grated ginger
- 1 tsp horseradish
- 1 tsp sea salt

Optional: 2 Tbsp hempseeds

- Sushi wrap = nori sheets
- Soy sauce = ¼ cup Mrs. Bragg's Liquid Aminos

✓ Break parsnips; then pulse in food processor; add grated ginger and horseradish and pulse. Add salt and pulse until parsnips are finely chopped but not soupy. Be careful because the heat can cause that.

Optional: Fold in hemp seeds.

Rolling Sushi

✓ Place 3 Tbsp of "rice" on raw nori sheet. Place steamed carrots, slices of avocado, and sprigs of cilantro on top and then roll using bamboo sushi rolling mat or a kitchen towel. Rolling sushi is its own art form. I recommend looking on YouTube to get a visual on rolling. Search for rolling sushi with or without a bamboo mat, depending on your situation. Sushi can be dipped in Mrs. Bragg's instead of soy sauce, which contains gluten and is fermented, two things I recommend we all avoid.

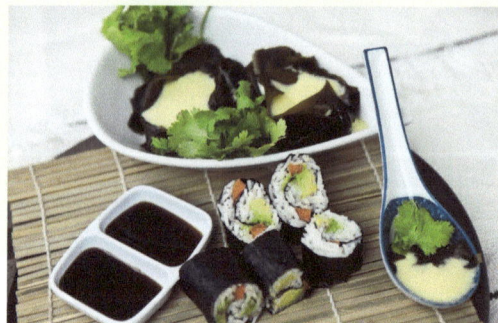

Seaweed Salad

- ◆ ½ cup wakame, arame, or hiziki
- ◆ ¼ cup filtered water
- ◆ ½ cup cilantro, finely chopped
- ◆ ¼ cup scallions, chopped

Optional: 1 crunchy pear, cubed

Salad dressing:

- ◆ Juice of half an orange
- ◆ ¼ cup raw tahini
- ◆ 1 tsp raw vinegar
- ◆ 2 Tbsp Mrs. Bragg's Liquid Aminos
- ◆ 1 tsp raw honey

✓ Soak seaweed in water and then toss with cilantro and scallions. Combine dressing ingredients in a bowl and pour over seaweed salad. Top with crunchy pear chunks.

FINAL THOUGHTS

Remember that you can add these recipes to your repertoire of recipes, one a week if you have to. Watch for improvements in your sense of well-being, ability to learn, performance, and physical health. Our problems, the places where we find ourselves stuck, are a manifestation of the gaps in our awareness. Nutrition is a powerful tool for helping to close those gaps. These recipes are all-natural and raw wherever possible to create a balance of vitamins, minerals, enzymes, and proteins your body needs to build itself at the highest level. Notice how much fiber is in these recipes. A daily bowel movement ensures your body has a fresh supply of nutrients, whereas old food in your system becomes toxic.

All over the world, there is hunger, and here in America, our cells also go without. We can make a new choice and eat "cell food" instead of constantly pushing our bodies out of balance with gluten, refined sugar, caffeine, low-grade dairy, high fructose corn syrup, and so forth—all of which are found in packaged foods. Learning to prepare food at home is the answer. This diet will balance your body so that you can find pleasure in going after a dream. Restaurant and processed foods rob us of the energy needed for reaching our highest potential because following our dreams takes all our might. Without the roller coaster of processed foods, you'll be sober enough to see a good opportunity to follow your dreams.

Living this way has made me wonderfully sober. I began wanting to expand myself, to be a speaker, an author, and a spiritual guide/life coach, and to confront my emotions and take risks that take my breath away. Pretty much, I wanted to do all things that both tantalize and terrify me. What if I try and fail? There has been so much fear in me. I have learned that, though meditation and being open to help from my divine, I can experience and release my fears and shift my consciousness, which brings exciting, new possibilities into my life and improves the quality of my existing relationships. Once you become aligned with your highest consciousness, you naturally begin to live in contribution to the lives of others and in a state of bliss, which is how God intended.

I invite you to make these healthy meals for yourself and your family. I invite you to meditate and pray. I invite you to embrace the diet and lifestyle necessary for you to live in bliss.

If we can do this, then we are finally listening to Hippocrates, long considered the father of modern medicine, who long ago left us sage advice: "Let food be thy medicine and medicine be thy food."

Thank you for listening to what I had to say. Be well.

By Esmeralda B. Fox